CAROL KRAKOWER, M.A. CCC-SLP

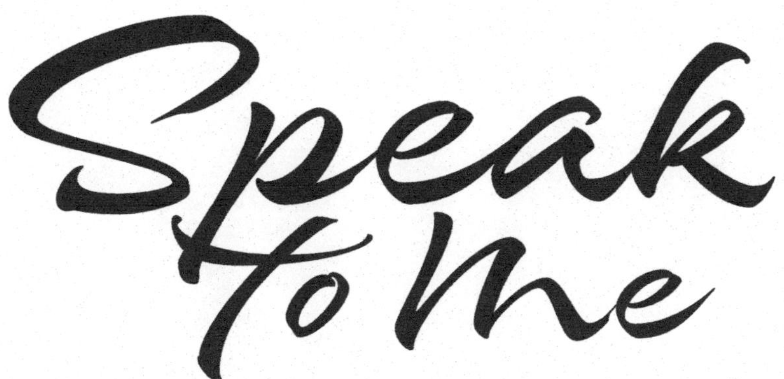

10 REASONS WHY YOUR CHILD IS NOT SPEAKING AS EXPECTED

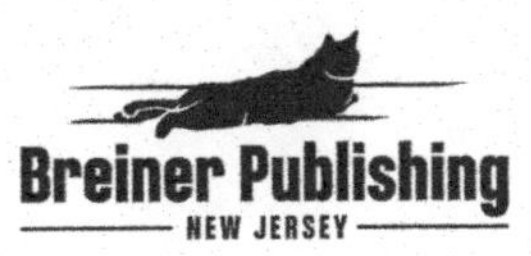

Breiner Publishing
NEW JERSEY

Contents

WHAT'S THE PROBLEM WITH ANDREW?

You are a parent or grandparent. You have a beautiful child. This child is wonderful is so many ways. But lately you are concerned that he is not speaking as well as you would expect at this age.

I am here help you. My name is Carol Krakower. I am the mother of five children, a grandmother and I have been a speech-language pathologist in private practice for many years. I have published therapy books for speech pathologists and have trained other speech pathologists. I want to guide you through a process so that you can understand what is normal in child speech development and what may indicate that your child needs assistance.

Let me tell you about a real child who came into my office.

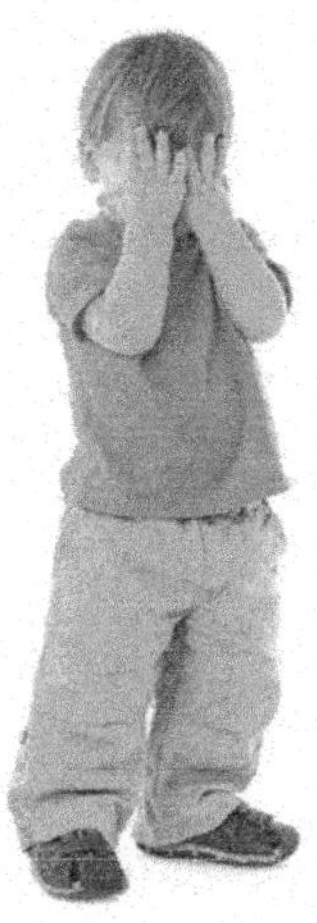

Andrew, just two years old, came into the speech therapy room without saying a word. He eyed me shyly from behind his mother's skirt. Andrew's mother said, "He used to say some words. Now he says nothing!" She pulled out her cell phone and showed me a video of Andrew repeating words to his mother: "mama, dada, wow." I nodded, yet I noticed on the video that Andrew's voice had an unusual resonance that made it difficult to understand what he was saying. I approached Andrew with a toy. He seemed to shrink when I started a game with him. Eventually, I was able to get him to warm up and play with toy cars. Then, I picked up a puppet and tried to get Andrew to teach the puppet to talk. I said a vowel sound, the puppet said the vowel sound, and Andrew just stared. No words. No imitations. I could see that Andrew had a "retrognathic profile" meaning that his chin receded. I put Nutella on a popsicle stick and licked it, then I made a Nutella pop for Andrew to lick. No luck. His mother said she had never seen Andrew stick out his tongue.

Andrew was making some gulping sounds. His mother said he made gulping sounds throughout the day. "Hmm" I thought, "audible swallowing is not normal." "Well," I said, "there are a few things we need to rule out before we diagnose a speech delay. I told her my recommendations. I will let you know in a little while how things turned out.

* * *

You know that all children are different. Albert Einstein is said to not have spoken until age 3, and he turned out to be a genius. Perhaps your child is the next Albert Einstein. But what if your child is struggling? The answer may not be so obvious.

Well-intentioned relatives may say to you, "Oh, remember little cousin Bobby. He wasn't talking at all on his third birthday, and then he suddenly began speaking and he's in third grade now and doing fine!" That may or may not be true, but it is only *one example*. Among all the children who are late talkers, a few may progress with no difficulties, but many more are not speaking *for a reason.* If your child is not speaking *for a reason,* you can help your child.

You may hear advice from people who feel that one size fits all. The mother down the street used straw and bubble exercises and her child began to speak. Then, of course, there are parents who post these types of ideas on their blogs with authority. Simply put, an internet diagnosis is about as reliable as the people posting the stories. Especially damaging are stories that one diagnosis *always includes* another diagnosis. Maybe it did for that parent's child, but not for every, or even for most, children.

If I hear one more story about how a special diet consisting of this special ingredient suddenly made a child start speaking, I will scream. This is simply not true. There may be some well-intentioned parents who began feeding their child a special ingredient at the same time the child responded to speech therapy, but the special ingredient did not *cause* the child to speak. Your child may have allergies to certain kinds of foods, and when you eliminate those foods, your child will feel better and be more open to learning. But no special ingredient makes a child speak.

Take all this type of advice with a grain of salt. Your child is unique. If you don't know *if* your child is actually struggling or delayed and if you don't know *why,* you may be wasting your time trying things that will not work.

Your concern may start in the pediatrician's office. When your child goes for well-visits, the pediatrician will screen your child for speech and language development. This is a screening; it is not an evaluation. A screening is designed to identify children who obviously have a developmental delay.

Typically, your pediatrician will ask at the 12-month checkup, "Is your child saying any words yet?" The average child at 12 months is saying a few words, usually "Dada," "Mama", perhaps a word for a grandparent and "baba" for a bottle. But that's the average child. It doesn't mean that a child who isn't saying a few words has a problem. He may say a few words in a few months and be perfectly within normal limits. Or he may not.

At the 24- month checkup, your pediatrician will ask how many words your child is saying and if he is putting two words together. This is a pass/fail screening. A child who does not have more than 50 words and is not putting two words together will be referred to a speech-language pathologist for a speech evaluation.

The problem is that many parents don't know how to answer this question. What is a word? Is "baba" for bottle a word? Suppose my child makes most animal sounds like "baa" and "moo"? Are they words? What about made-up words? Are they words? And what does it mean to "put two words together?" Does that mean "thank you" or "all done!" or does it mean that the child spontaneously says, "Daddy home!" If the pediatrician expresses concern, you will probably go to the internet to do some research.

You may wonder: Is it my fault?

In all my years of doing speech evaluations, I have noticed that most parents feel some degree of guilt. This may not be your first child and you may be wondering why the first child spoke so well at this age and this child does not. Is it because one is a boy and one is a girl? Is it because one was "stimulated" more than the other? Parents with one child may still have the feeling that if he had received more stimulation, he would talk. This has been convoluted from research studies showing that children who receive virtually no stimulation have delays. Yes, if your child was left unattended for most hours every day in his crib, there would be developmental consequences. However, most children who are loved and cared for will begin to speak on their own. If your child is not speaking there may be a struggle within the child.

Parents are also afraid that their child might not be "smart." Although language development is tied to cognitive development, there are children who are *very* smart, but who have structural, muscular, motor planning, language or auditory struggles that show up in a speech or language delay.

When a parent brings a child to my office for a speech evaluation, especially the first child in the family, there is often some difference of opinion in the family about whether an evaluation is necessary. Sometimes it is a grandparent who tells the parent that there is cause for concern. Very often I see a mother who is worried, but a father who is angry that anyone who would "say something is wrong with my kid.

Sometimes parents feel guilty that they didn't recognize the speech difficulty *sooner*. It's not aways easy to know if your child is on target, or just immature or struggling. What's important now is that you find out how your child is really doing, and address any difficulty you discover.

Communication difficulties in childhood are relatively common. Nearly one in twelve children ages 3–17 has a disorder related to voice, speech, language or swallowing. Boys are more likely than girls to be affected, and preschool children have the highest level of communication disorders – almost 11 percent. If one in twelve children in the United States has a speech, language, voice or swallowing difficulty, that means that over 6 million children have speech difficulty.

Some people with communication difficulties in childhood have been known to go on and become famous for their speaking abilities. Actor James Earl Jones is famous for his voice as Darth Vader in *Star Wars, and* the voice that says "This is CNN." He had a severe stutter as a child and seldom spoke.

What if I just let my child "grow out of it?"

If your child cannot easily communicate with others, the child may face some likely consequences. Your child may experience frustration and tantrums. Your child could be made fun of by other children. If your child is having difficulty hearing sounds in words, he will probably have difficulty learning to read.

Learning to speak is a natural process. Most children do it on their own. That does not mean that learning to speak is not a *complex process.* Learning to speak and use language involves coordinating a symphony of sub-skills. This book will teach you what is required to understand language and speak to that you can identify what sub-skills might be a struggle for your child. Sometimes anxious parents bring their child for an evaluation and I say at the end of the evaluation, "Don't worry. Your child is within normal limits." Other times, I say "Yes, your child is struggling and here is the reason and here is what we plan to do to help your child communicate." I can't tell you how often parents tell me that they are glad to get a diagnosis. Their relief comes from finding a solution to the nagging feeling about their child's speech delay.

I will take you through the stages of what I look for when a child enters my office. This does not substitute for a speech evaluation, but it will point you in the right direction.

I'm sure you're wondering, what happened to Andrew?

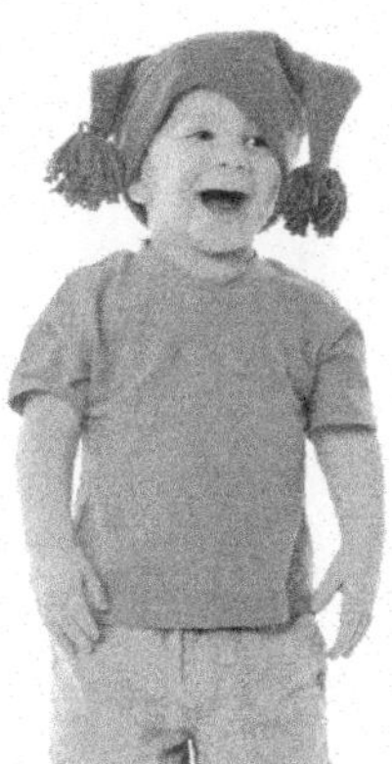

I referred Andrew to an ENT and audiologist. It turns out, Andrew was hearing virtually nothing. Andrew's ears were so clogged he needed tubes, which were scheduled immediately.

I also referred him to a maxillofacial surgeon for a suspected posterior tongue tie. Although Andrew did not have a "heart-shaped" tongue so typical of tongue tie, there were other signs. The oral surgeon said it was one of the worst cases of tongue tie he had ever seen. Andrew had a frenectomy, where a surgeon cuts the membrane under his tongue to free his tongue for greater movement.

A few months later, after speech therapy, Andrew was laughing and speaking happily. Once his structural issues were resolved through surgery and then speech therapy, he was able to progress normally.

Does speech therapy work? Yes! It is never one-size-fits-all. Speech therapy is an educated, step-by-step approach targeting the child's specific challenges with researched techniques.

My goal is to provide you with good information mixed with years of experience. You will find out the difference between "typical" speech and "normal" speech. You will learn about possible reasons why a child is not speaking. You will learn when a child's speech is developmentally appropriate and when it is not. You will learn when to seek help for your child. As a parent, wany to feel that you have learned and done everything you can for your precious child. My goal is to empower you and your child with the knowledge you need.

PART I

Language

HOW IS LANGUAGE LEARNED?

How is "language" different from "speech?"

Speech is talking. You need to coordinate breath with vocal cords and use the mouth, jaw, tongue and vocal tract in a very precise and coordinated way to say words that others understand.

Underlying speech is language.

Language is a system of words and symbols that convey meaning. Language can be written, spoken or signed. Despite the fact that language is incredibly complex, the typical child will progress along developmental steps to speak in an adult-like manner by kindergarten. I will discuss five aspects of language.

Semantics

The vocabulary of the language is called *semantics* by linguists. When you read a board book to your baby and ask him to point to the horse, you are teaching him semantics.

Morphology and Syntax

Besides the words themselves, languages have rules about how words can be put together. This is the grammar of the language, called *morphology* and *syntax*. For example, *dog* means one particular animal and *dogs* means two or more of the same animal.

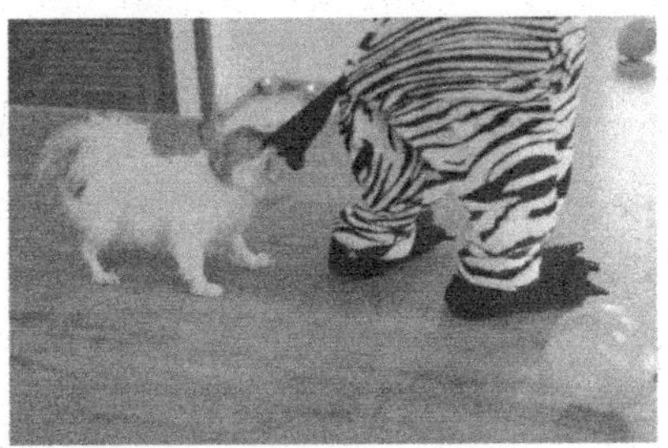 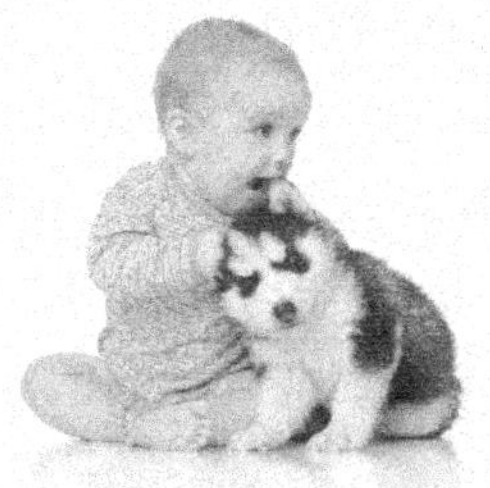

If a child says *doggy bite,* it means that the doggy bit the child but *bite doggy* means that the child bit the dog! Your child is learning how to assemble sentences for correct meaning. A child learning English must say *Daddy jumped in the pool* instead of *Jumped pool Daddy.*

Syntax can be quite complex. Yet, by age five, most children understand language rules well enough to be able to select the correct picture to this sentence: *The boy who is sitting under the big tree is eating a banana.* They will discard the picture of a boy sitting under a little tree, they will discard the picture of the boy sitting under a big tree without a banana and they will discard a picture of a boy standing under a big tree eating a banana.

Phonology

Your child is learning to correctly produce the sounds of his native language. This is called *phonology* and each discrete sound is called a *phoneme.* Although there are only 26 letters in the English language, there are 44 phonemes in American English, 24 consonant sounds and about 20 vowel sounds. (The number of vowel sounds can change depending upon accent.) Consider the letter "e." Now think of baseball player Derek Jeter. The first two *e's* in his name are short /e/ and then we have a long *ee,* of *Je-* and his name ends with a vocalic /r/ *er.* That one /e/ is three distinct sounds in just one name!

Pragmatics

Pragmatic language is understanding the rules of social language. One of the first aspects of pragmatic language that a baby learns is turn-taking. Baby may blow a raspberry, and then Mommy blows a raspberry back at him. Baby smiles, realizing that this is a back-and-forth. He blows a raspberry back at Mommy. It is more than just a game; it is language learning. He is learning to maintain eye contact with a communication partner and take turns.

Pragmatic language also involves learning to wave *hi* and *bye-bye* in appropriate social situations. Later, the child will learn that when someone asks a question, he expects a response and that that no one will listen to a long monologue.

Pragmatics also includes understanding *appropriate vocal volume*. How many young children must be reminded to use "indoor voice" and not "outdoor voice?" It includes using the correct *tone of voice*. Some tones of voice are considered "fresh." It may be okay to shout to your friend in the park, "Hey! Gimme a cookie!" but it would not be okay to shout to Grandma at the dinner table, "Hey! Gimme a cookie!"

A typical child learns to use the intonation patterns of her native language to convey meaning. This is called *prosody*.

For example, if she said *Daddy jumped in the pool* and her pitch went *down* at the end of the sentences, she is telling you what Daddy did: he jumped in the pool.

Daddy jumped in the   *pool.*
                          pool.   *Daddy jumped in the*

If her pitch goes *up* at the end of the sentence, she is asking you a question: *Daddy jumped in the pool?* A baby learns prosody even before she has real words. Have you had a "conversation" with your baby in which it *sounds like* she is speaking because her babble has the rhythm and intonation of English?

Gestures help a child learn language. When you extend your open palm and say, "Give it to Mommy," the baby learns what *give* means. Some parents are afraid that using gestures with a baby will hinder his language development, but this is not so. This is why finger-plays are so appealing to toddlers – the gestures of the itsy-bitsy spider climbing help the child to understand the meaning of the rhyme! Of course, if a child communicates *primarily* in gestures by about 18 months, there would be concern that he is not using words, too.

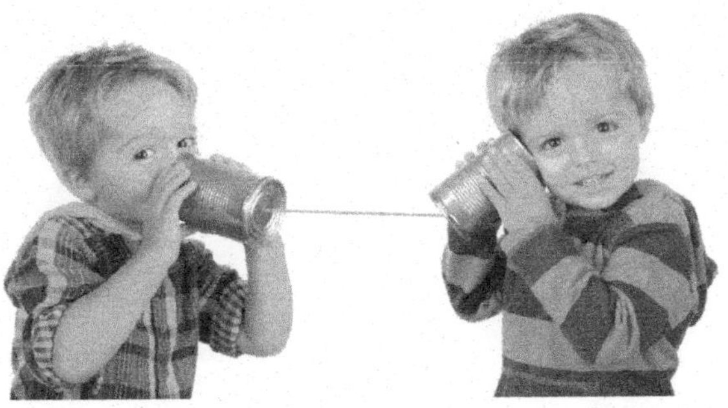

Receptive and Expressive Language

The child learns to use all these aspects of language for both *receptive language,* or what he understands, and *expressive language,* or how he uses language to communicate. A child with a good receptive language ability understands words and language on an age-appropriate level. If he hears two adults talking together about how today might be a good day to go out to the park, he may run and get his coat. He understands what is said, even though it wasn't said directly to him, and he is anticipating that he will need his coat! A child with a good expressive language ability is able to form sentences and ask and answer questions on an age-appropriate basis. He may be able to enter Grandma's house and ask, "Where's the kitty? I will find him!"

Do children understand more than they are able to express?

In typically developing children, yes. A child who understands about 50 words may only be saying one to five words.

In the next chapter, I will discuss the typical stages of language development for most children. These is important to know so that you can identify if your child has a speech or language learning delay.

TYPICAL LANGUAGE DEVELOPMENT

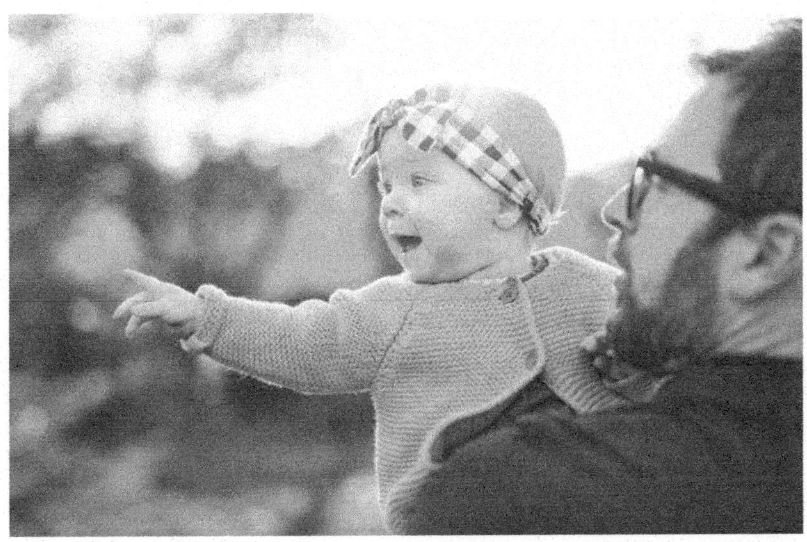

It's important to understand that there are developmental stages of speech and language development and it begins at birth.

In 1973, speech-language theorist Roger Brown published a book entitled "A First Language: The Early Stages." Brown identified definable stages of language development that are used today. Speech pathologists use these stages to identify which children are progressing on a normal course of language learning and which children are struggling.

0-3 months

Incredibly, a newborn baby can turn to you when you speak and smiles when he hears your voice. Research has shown that a three-day-old infant can recognize his mother's voice over others and shows preference for human voices over other sounds. A newborn baby under three months will stop his activity and listen closely to an unfamiliar voice. He responds to comforting tones whether the voice is familiar or not. He can discriminate speech sounds from environmental sounds. By two months, he can follow another person's gaze and by 3 months can shift his gaze to follow an adult's gaze.

4-6 months

By 4-6 months, the baby is interested in all sounds and can be fascinated by squeaky toys or musical mobiles.

7-12 months

Seven to twelve months is an exciting and fun time as the baby now listens to you when you speak to him, turns and looks at your face when you call his name and discovers the fun of games like "peek a boo." He is also learning the meaning of some words, like *Dada* or the name of a toy or pet. He can follow some simple directions with gestures, such as "give it to Mama." The baby is now babbling to himself and others. He is practicing sounds and words and developing intonation patterns, amusing his parents by doing things like yelling at the cat angrily in his own language! By the first birthday, a typical child has a few words that parents recognize, usually the names of people or objects close to him: *Mama, Dada, Nana, baba* for a bottle or perhaps a word for the family pet.

After the first birthday, most babies learn words rapidly. Most babies say only a few words on their first birthday, but the average toddler says about 260 words by the second birthday.

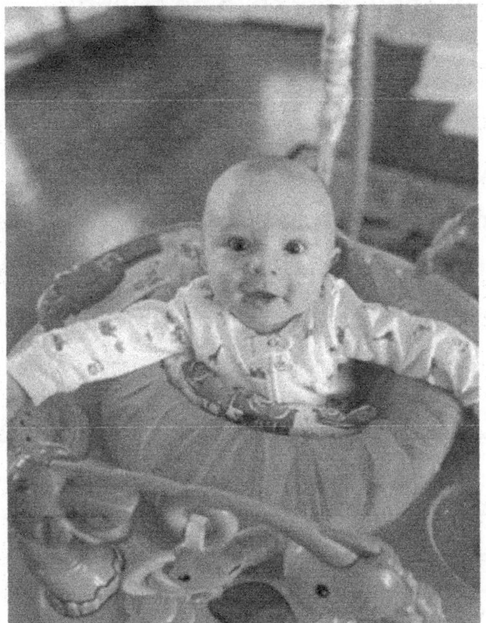

What is a word?

Most parents don't know how to answer this question. Is "baba" for bottle a word? What about animal sounds like "baa" and "moo"? Are they words? What about made-up words?

For a speech pathologist, a word is an actual word that other people can understand to mean the intended item. If your child points to a stuffed bunny and says, "bun-bun" I would accept that as a word because it is close to the actual word bunny, so close, in fact, that I know what it is. If he points to it and says, "gee," I would not consider that a word.

Consider it a word when it is said *consistently*, meaning that he always says this word for this thing; *independently*, meaning that he can say the word without coaching and *intentionally*, meaning he is trying to communicate with the word.

How many words should my child be saying?

The short answer is that there is a range of how many words a child should be saying, depending upon whether you look at what the average child does or look at what ninety percent of children do. The average child is far ahead of the measure of what ninety percent of children do. Of course, some children will have more words than the average child.

Here is a chart of what the numbers of words the *average* child says and the number of words *ninety percent* of children have by age:

Age	Average child	90% of children
12 months	5	1
18 months	50	10
24 months	260	50
36 months	Over 1,000	250

12 months

At twelve months, the *average* child will be saying about five words. Ninety percent of children will be saying at least one word. At eighteen months, the *average* child will say 50 words, and ninety percent of children will say 10 words. Most eighteen-month-old children are not yet combining two words.

Besides just words, what should you be looking for in your one-year-old? The typical one-year-old uses some gestures to request, such as reaching towards his bottle and pushing away something he is refusing. By eighteen months, he may use gestures to direct attention to himself or someone else.

He is learning to listen to simple board books and points to pictures of things in a familiar book when you name them. He is also learning to point to body parts. The first body parts will be major ones, such as head, feet, hand, and eyes. Later, he will be able to point to his elbow, his knee, or his eyebrow. The typical one-year-old increases his vocabulary every month.

His words become clearer as he gains more fine-motor movement for speech. When a baby first begins to say a word such as "dada" he moves his entire jaw and tongue up to make the /d/ sound. Later, he is able to elevate his tongue to his palate to make the /d/ sound to say dada.

In our office, we often see parents of 12–14-month-old children who are worried that the child has very few words. If the child has communicative ability, understands language on an age-appropriate level, and does not have something that would prevent progress, such as a tongue tie or a hearing loss, I would tell the parent that the child seems to be progressing *normally*.

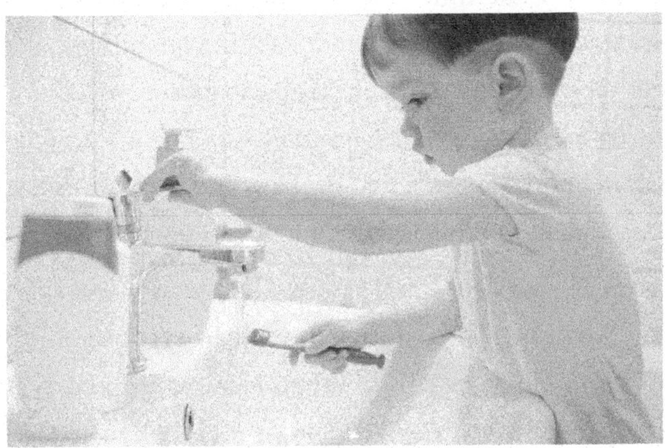

Typical Language Development in a 2-year-old

By the second birthday, the *average* child will have about two hundred sixty words, including action words, and will be combining them into two-word combinations. By this we mean two words that, put together, form a concept, such as *puppy sick* or *more juice*. We don't mean memorized two-word phrases, like *thank you* and *all gone*. Ninety percent of children will have over fifty words. If your baby is not saving fifty words on his second birthday and is not combining two words, it is certainly time to find out why.

By the second birthday, the typical child is combining words into a complete thought. Many of her words will be action words, such as *run, eat, jump.* She may be saying things like *more juice, horsie go, daddy home, push truck, water hot.*

She can react to things with words like *wow!* and *uh-oh!* She will have social words, such as *please* and *thank you.* Her words may not yet be pronounced clearly, but may be said consistently. For example, she may consistently say *doe* for "go" and the family knows that she means "go."

She will start to ask questions, such as "Where ball?" "What's that? and can answer simple questions. She is beginning to use pronouns, such as *you, I,* or *her.*

She is able to use inflection to convey statements and questions: *Daddy home. Daddy home?* She is understanding quantities, and knows the difference between *sock* and *socks.* She is able to follow two commands, such as *go into the bathroom and get your toothbrush.* She is learning basic concepts, such as *hot* and *cold, stop* and *go.* Now the family understands what the child is saying, although her speech may not yet be clear to strangers.

This is an age for very simple stories, songs and fingerplays. She will enjoy hearing the same songs, stories and fingerplays over and over again. She can also learn words by doing. When I evaluate a two-year-old's language ability, I present a toy train and show the child how to blow the whistle. I am looking to see if the child can imitate the action of blowing the whistle. Later in the evaluation, I will ask her to blow the whistle without showing her again to determine if she learned the words *blow the whistle.*

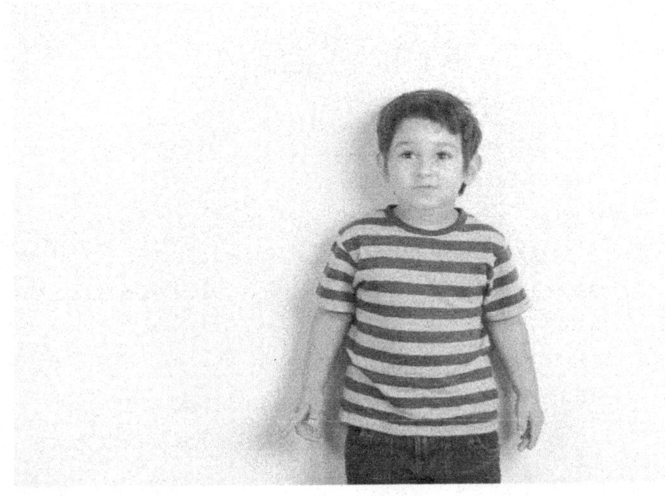

Typical Language Development After Age 3

By the third birthday, the average child will have over a thousand words and will be combining them into sentences. Ninety percent of children will have about two hundred fifty words.

Now the typical child understands simple *who, what* and *where* questions. Sentences become longer and the child talks about things that have happened away from home, such as pre-school, friends, outings and interesting experiences. Speech is usually fluent and clear people outside of the family can understand what your child is saying most of the time. By the time the typical child is five and a half, he can tell a story, engage in conversation and says all speech sounds clearly.

How's My Child Doing?
Language Learning milestones of the typical child

MY 1-YEAR-OLD	Looks when you point
	Recognizes his name
	Says two or three words
	Recognizes words for familiar people and items, such as Mama, a favorite toy, a bottle, a pet
	Responds to simple words and phrases, such as *come here, give it to Mama, no*
	Plays games with you, such as peek-a-boo and *so big!*
	Uses gestures, such as waving bye-bye, shaking head *no*
	Babbles and talks to himself in what sounds like his native language, albeit without real words
MY 2-YEAR-OLD	Has a vocabulary of about 260 words
	Some of the vocabulary words are action words, such as *eat, run, fall down, go*
	Points to body parts when asked
	Understands *where* and *who* questions, such as *where are your shoes?* or *who is that?*
	Listens to stories, fingerplays, rhymes
	Points to pictures named in a book, such as *point to the bear, point to the bird*
	Can name familiar pictures in a book
	Puts two words together in unique combinations, such as *Daddy home* or *puppy sick*
MY 3-YEAR-OLD	Can follow two-step directions: *go upstairs and find your teddy bear*
	Understands new words quickly
	Understands opposites, such as *stop-go, little-big, up-down*
	Has a word for all the familiar people and things in his life
	Regularly uses action words, such as *walk, eat, jump, run, swim, drive*
	Talks about something that is not in the room
	Talks when engaging in pretend play, such as pretending to talk on the phone
	Understands and uses *in, on, under*
	Asks *why* questions
	Speaks in sentences

How's My Child Doing?
Language Learning milestones of the typical child

MY 4-YEAR-OLD	Can identify shapes, such as *square, circle, triangle*
	Can identify colors, such as *red, blue, green*
	Understands relationship words for family members, such as *grandmother, brother, uncle*
	Answers *who, what, where, when* and *how* questions
	Can rhyme words, such as *cat-hat, bear-chair*
	Use pronouns *I, you, me, we* and *they*
	Uses plurals, such as *two cats, all my toys*
	Talks about what happened during the day
MY 5-YEAR-OLD	Understands words for order, such as *first this happened, next this happened and last this happened*
	Understands time concepts, such as *yesterday, today, tomorrow*
	Understands most of what is said at home and in school
	Identifies letters and numbers
	Tells a short story

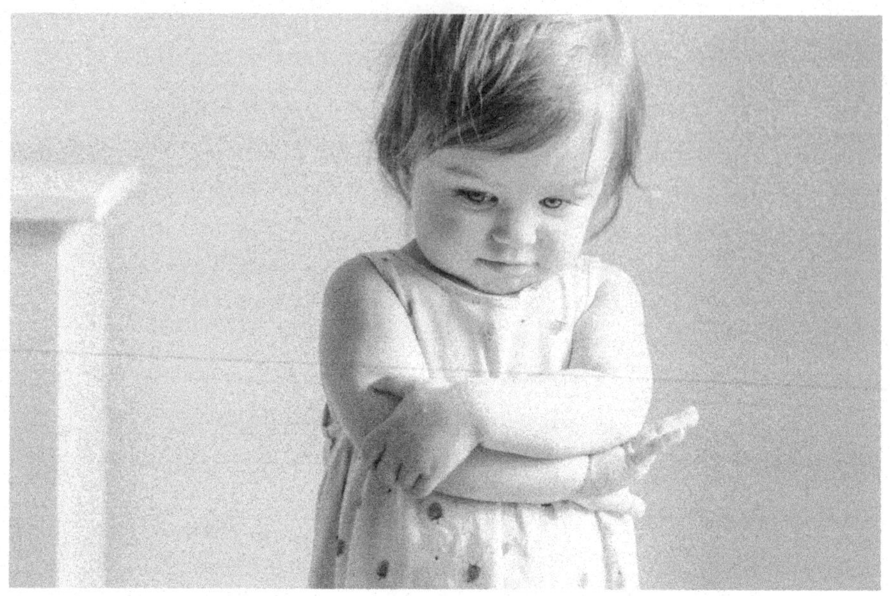

Why Doesn't My Child Listen to Me?

Suppose you point and tell your 2-year-old to fetch her shoes. To understand you and do what you ask, your child must

* Be attuned to you with joint attention

* clearly hear what you are saying

* understand the words you are speaking.

If she struggles with any one of these three sub-skills, she will not fetch her shoes.

JOINT ATTENTION & COMMUNICATIVE INTENT

After reading the previous chapter, if you have determined that your child's language is delayed, it may indicate that your child is struggling. One of the first indications of a struggle is a child who does not appear to pay attention to his parent.

In this chapter and the next two chapters, I will explain three common reasons why a child may not appear to listen to you.

Reason #1: My child lacks joint attention and communicative intent

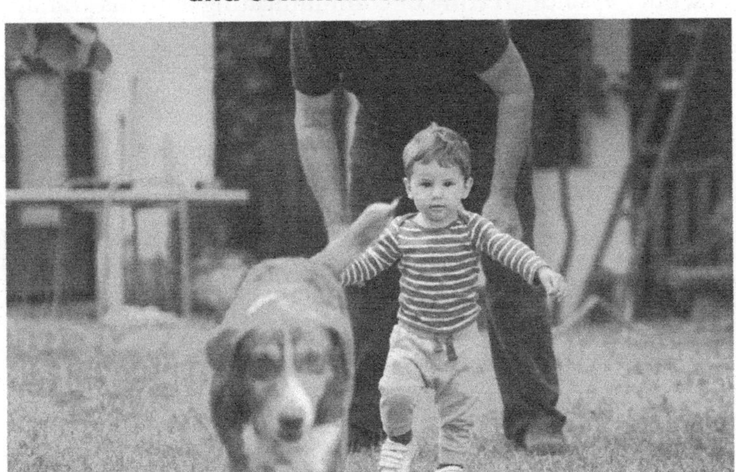

Noah's grandmother brought him into our speech office for an evaluation. She was concerned that, when he comes to her home, he says "Grandma and Pop Pop's house" but then brushes right past Grandma and Pop Pop and

does not greet them. He maneuvers straight to his favorite things. She said that Noah is able to request things by naming the item and saying please, such as "Cookie please.," but it is as if he has a magic lantern and when he declares what he wants, the object magically appears. He is not looking at his grandmother to request cookies from her. During the evaluation, it was very difficult to get Noah's attention. He did not respond to his name being called. He said "boat" and "truck" when wanting those toys. Several times, when he attempted to try a new toy and got stuck, he cried "Help, please" to no one in particular. Noah was very self-directed. He would not do anything requested of him, would not point to a picture or repeat a word. He was intent on doing his own thing.

What is communicative intent?

In a speech pathologist's eyes, Noah may be saying words, but he is not deliberately communicating a message to another person through eye gaze, gestures or speech. He is identifying Grandma and Pop Pop's house when he arrives, but he is not greeting or communicating with his grandparents. Communicative intent is the use of eye contact, gestures, facial expressions and, eventually, spoken words to deliver a message to another person.

In typical children the desire to communicate with other people is innate: even if they have impaired hearing, they will communicate through eye gaze, pointing, even vocalizations. Some children, though, do not understand that they must communicate with *other people*.

Noah is saying words, but it is self-talk.

What is joint attention?

Joint attention is the ability of two people to attend to the same object or action. One person calls the other's attention to the object or action by pointing to it or gazing at it. The other person follows the pointing or eye gaze and they both know that they are seeing the same thing.

How do communicative intent and joint attention develop?

During the first months of life, infants and their caregivers typically communicate face to face. Mother looks at baby with interest and love; baby learns to intentionally return her gaze and eventually, return her smile or coo. This is an example of communicative intent.

As the baby gets older, he begins to interacts with objects in the environment. The baby may call mother's attention to an object and look to see whether the mother sees the same thing. This is an example of joint attention. In this picture, the baby looks at the puppy, then checks his parent's attention to the puppy. This is an example of developing joint attention.

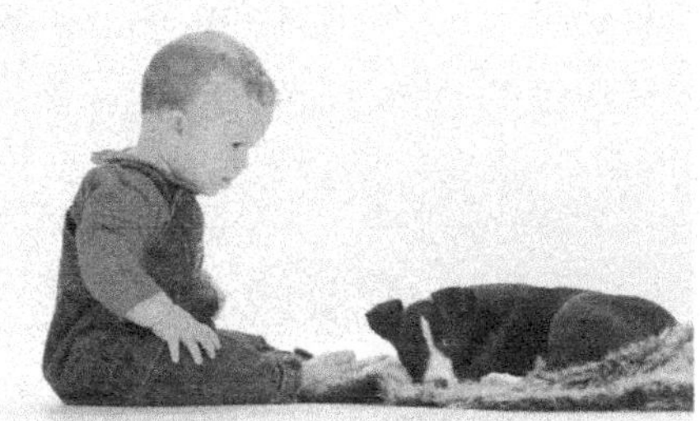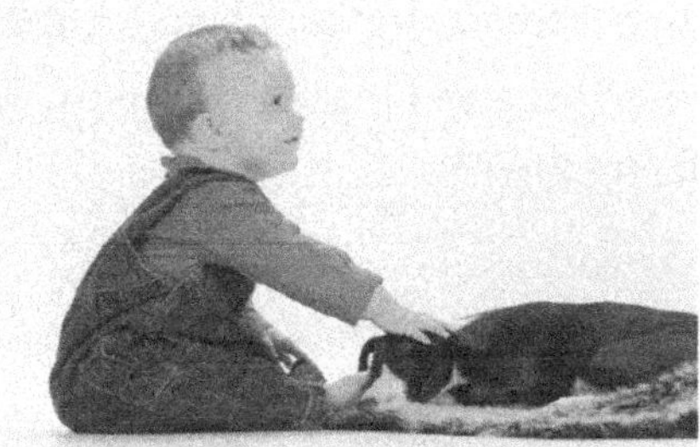

In typical development, joint attention skills emerge in the following order:

Between 6 and 12 months, babies begin to check their parent's reaction to objects or actions in their environment. The baby might look at a puppy, then at Daddy and then back to the puppy, suggesting that he knows that Daddy sees the puppy, too. There is an understanding between Baby and Daddy that they are both paying attention to the puppy. At first, these glances might be fleeting, but by about 12 months, babies become quite intentional about checking out another's reaction to something in the environment.

At about 10 months, most babies begin "showing." They will hold up an object to show it to another person.

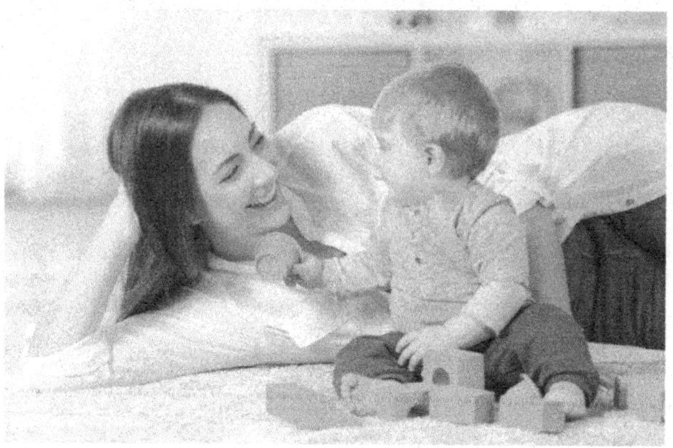

By the first birthday, most babies can follow another person's gaze to an item or another person. The child is able to know that you are seeing something and if she gazes in the same direction, she will know what you are looking at.

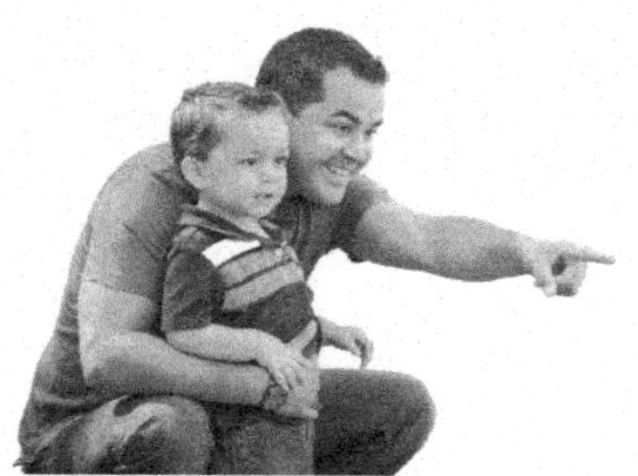 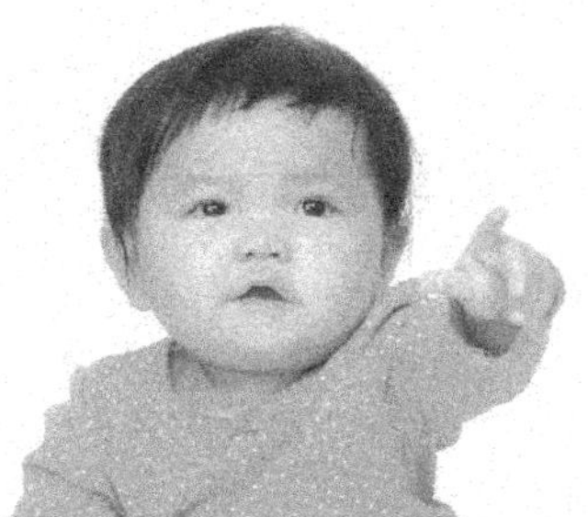

By 14 months, most babies can look in the direction in which someone points. By 16 months, they can point to objects themselves to communicate with others. Babies point to make requests, such as *I want that cookie* and share experiences, such as *See the funny dog?*

In summary, joint attention means that your child joins you or engages you to both pay attention to the same thing. Your child should be pointing to an object, then looking at you to determine if you understand what she is pointing at, and then back to the object. This back-and-forth is an important component of joint attention. A child who points at an object but does not look up to see if you notice is only engaging in wishful thinking: if I point, maybe it will come my way. How different that is from looking at Mommy and pointing to indicate "I'm pointing to *that*, Mommy. That one over there! See it? Can you help me get it?"

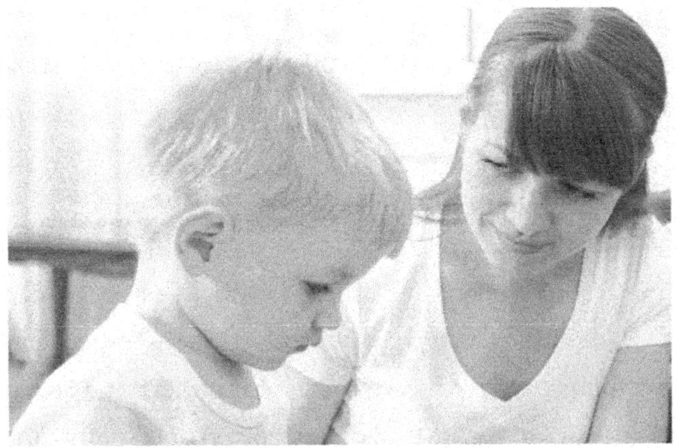

This is James. James is a 3-and-a-half-year-old boy who made little eye contact with me during the speech evaluation. In school, he enjoys parallel play but little interaction with other children. He does not interact with his younger sister at home. James is able to name objects with single words. He is able to repeat words and sentences but not yet able to form sentences of his own. When he wants something, he takes his mother's hand and silently leads her to what he wants. His mother reports that when he got his finger stuck in a shopping cart, rather than alert his mother to his predicament, he took his mother's hand and put it on top of his stuck finger to get it loosened. Because James does not have the intention of communicating with others, he is also missing opportunities for joint attention.

Why is joint attention important?

Joint attention is the back-and-forth that is necessary to engage in communication with others. Without it, a child such as Noah may talk without any expectation of being answered and may not answer when spoken to. With it, a child such as James does not get help when he needs help. Joint attention is a social skill.

A toddler with limited joint attention may have difficulty acquiring a broad range of developmental skills including learning how to communicate with other people.

Is lack of joint attention and communicative intent associated with autism?

When a child's joint attention is consistently limited or absent, we become concerned about autism. Children diagnosed with autism often have trouble following gestures, eye gaze, and/or using words to communicate. Although a child with autism may point to something he wants, he often does not look to his parent to see if the parent understands what he wants. A child with autism often won't follow when someone points. Although he may use many words to label things, some of which may be quite advanced, he usually does not communicate *with others.* A little boy came into my office recently and was playing with toy food. He was able to identify even the unusual fruit, such as pineapple and kiwi, but he wasn't showing me the fruit; he was labeling each item to himself.

How do I know if my child is struggling with communicative intent and joint attention?

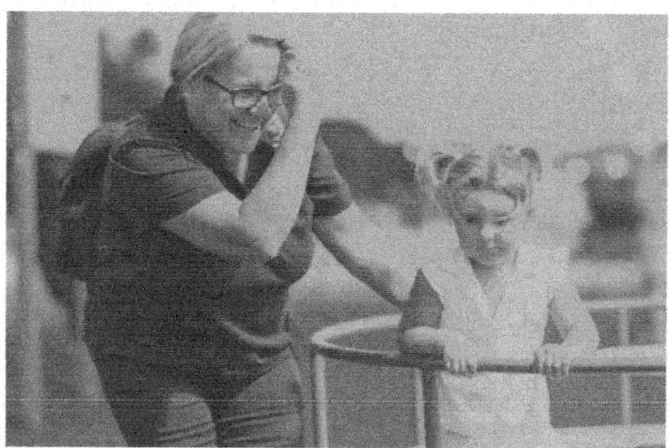

Emma is a 3-year-old girl who recently came into our office. Emma's mother listed 100 words that Emma says currently. She is not yet speaking in sentences. She does not yet call her parents Mama or Dada, but she can repeat those words. In fact, Emma can repeat anything that is said to her, but doesn't form her own sentences. Emma has memorized some automatic words, such as "Open!" and "All done!" and "up!" but she does not look at her parents when she makes these requests. Emma can imitate actions done by another, such as pushing a button on a toy. When Emma needs to request something from her parent, she grabs her mother's hand and brings her to the object. She does not look at her mother when she does this.

A child who has difficulty with communicative intent will often repeat what she hears on the television, or on a favorite recording. This is called *echolalia.* Although the child can repeat words, she is only parroting what she has heard before. She is not able to answer a simple question. When asked a question, the child will often repeat the last word of the question. Do you want cookies? *Cookies.* Shall we take a bath? *Bath.* Often times, the child will remember routines, such as bath time, and she will run upstairs to fetch bath toys after dinner, but is not communicating with her parents; she anticipates a familiar routine. In order to move a child from echolalia to intent, it is important for the parent to work with a speech pathologist to create situations in which the child must learn to communicate.

Usually, a parent has an uneasy feeling that her child is not communicating with her. The child may never answer to her name, but continues to "do her own thing." She appears to ignore others most of the time. Things need to be her idea or she's not interested. Adults may have to work pretty hard to get and keep this child's attention. Often, a parent worries that inadequate parenting causes this lack of attention. There are many well-loved and well-cared for children who do not show joint attention and communicative intent despite their parents' best efforts! It can be difficult for a parent to recognize that it is the child who is struggling.

To make parenting all the more challenging, children with joint attention difficulties may exhibit tantrums because they feel that things that they want should magically appear. If the child desires cheese, she stands by the refrigerator and assumes Mom knows her desire. When cheese does not show up, she tantrums.

A child without joint attention skills may not know how to play with other children. She may be too physical with other children, such as biting or hitting other children, or pushing another child out of the way, unaware that the child will not like that.

Most children gradually develop more mature ways to gain attention from others. Although a typical child at 12 months may fuss or cry when she wants something, by the toddler years the child will look toward, point, or lead parents to what she wants. A toddler with limited joint attention will still just cry.

How can a speech pathologist help my child with communicative intent and joint attention?

A speech pathologist will develop an individual plan to help your child develop communicative intent. One method often used is putting preferred items, such as toys and books, in clear plastic bins that are difficult to open on a shelf so that the child cannot reach it. The child must learn to communicate what he wants each day. Often, the child will not know that he must use a word and communicate it to his parent to get the toy. The Picture Exchange System is a temporary tool used to teach the child to communicate with words. There is a picture for each of his toys and favorite foods. The child has access to the pictures of the items, and learns to choose a picture, bring it to his parent, look at his parent and say the word in order to get the food or toy. These methods are not designed to be permanent, but to gradually help the child learn to inter-act with others to communicate.

To improve joint attention with your child, get down to the level of his face to make eye contact with him. For example, kneel down so that your eyes are across from his eyes, and tell him, "Come. It's time to go."

The most important recommendation I can make for parents of a child who is struggling with joint attention is to get professional assistance. Begin by discussing the concerns with your pediatrician. Ask for a referral for a developmental assessment. A developmental pediatrician can assess your child for developmental delays. Get a speech/language evaluation. Getting help early is especially crucial since he won't "grow out of it." Intervention in the pre-school and toddler years can significantly improve your child's joint attention that is so critical for communication.

Checklist for Parents: How's My Child Doing?
Source: ASHA Social Communication Benchmarks, developed from information from Gard, Gilman & Gorman (1993) and Russell (2007)

DOES YOUR BABY UP TO 12 MONTHS OLD:

Prefer to look at a human face and human eyes

Prefer to listen to a person's voice

Look around when hearing a voice to see who is speaking

Differentiate between tones of voice (*i.e.*, angry voice or friendly voice)

Smile back when smiled at

Follow caregiver's gaze

take turns vocalizing with caregiver

Vocalize to get attention

Demonstrate joint attention skills, checking the face of the person with whom the baby is inter-acting

Request by gesturing and/or vocalizing

Play simple interactive games, such as peek-a-boo

DOES YOUR 12–18-MONTH-OLD:

Show objects to others

Request by pointing and verbalizing

Try to get attention by vocalizing

Say *bye-bye*

Protest by shaking head *no*

Look at the person who is speaking

Demonstrate sympathy, empathy or sharing non-verbally

DOES YOUR 18–24-MONTH-OLD:

Use single words to communicate with others *i.e., Puppy!*

Use single words or paired words to command *i.e., more juice!*

Use single words to indicate possession *i.e., mine!*

Use single words to express problems *i.e., Help please!* or gain attention *i.e., look!* and looks at the person to whom he is speaking

Use pronouns *I, me, you, my* and *mine*

Take turns in conversation

Understand the topic being discussed and stay on topic. For example, if you say, "We are going to the park" will your child respond with something about the park, such as "swings!"

DOES YOUR 24–36-MONTH-OLD:

Engage in short dialogues

Introduce a new topic or change topics *i.e., Look, Mama! Puppy!*

Express emotion

Start to use language in an imaginative way

Relate his own experiences *i.e. I fell down!*

Begin to use descriptive detail *i.e., scary monster!*

Use attention-getting words *i.e., help me!*

Clarify and ask for clarification *i.e., not Jack's dog, my dog!*

Use some politeness terms i.e., *juice, please!*

AUDITORY DISORDERS

Reason #2: My child cannot hear well.

You may be saying: "I don't need to read this chapter. My child passed the newborn hearing screening in the hospital. The pediatrician screens my child during a check-up, and except for a few ear infections, he's been fine."

Did you know that your child must not only hear *well enough to learn,* but must also *learn* to hear? Requirements for learning to hear are stringent. The reality is that you often *can't tell* if your child is hearing *well enough.* If you child is not hearing well, he doesn't know that he could possibly hear better, and he can't tell you. Many times, we evaluate children in our office whose difficulty stems from undetected hearing difficulty. You'd better read this chapter.

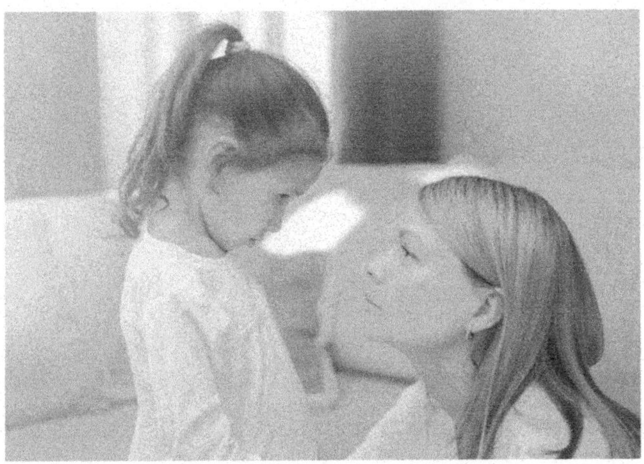

This is Riley. When she came into our office for a speech evaluation, it was very difficult to understand what she was saying because she was distorting most of her speech sounds. Her parents complained that she seldom listens to them and wondered if her hearing was "selective." As a speech pathologist, I know that distorted sounds are often a sign of poor hearing. Many preschoolers make sound substitutions, such as saying "wittle wamb" for "little lamb." But a sound distortion means the sound does not match any sound in English. When I hear this, I always suspect that child had, or currently has, a hearing loss. I asked her parents to bring her to a pediatric audiologist to check her hearing first. Her father balked. "She has never had a hearing problem." Well, two weeks later, Riley was back – with tubes in her ears! It turns out, she had a lot of fluid in her ears, but never complained, so her parents never knew!

We don't hear with our ears.

Auditory system

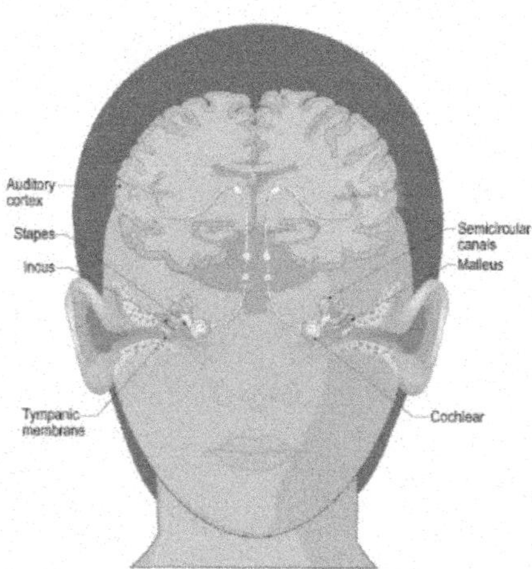

The outer ear captures and detects vibrations. The vibrations pass into the ear drum through the middle ear, where three tiny bones, the *ossicles*, detect the vibrations and pass those vibrations to the inner ear. The inner ear is lined with fluid and tiny hair cells, which pass these vibrations through the auditory nerve to the temporal lobe of the brain.

Not all sound comes through the ears. We also conduct vibrations through the bones in our head, and these vibrations are also passed into the inner ear and then the auditory nerve.

When the vibrations are received by the brain, it is perceived as "sound."

Hearing is as much perceptual as physical. Sounds must be organized in the brain before they can be interpreted. A baby must *learn* to hear.

We hear sounds in the brain.

You may not be aware of your child's hearing loss. The screening at the pediatrician's office is not enough when there is a speech or language issue. An evaluation by a pediatric audiologist is a necessary first step.

Before I can make a diagnosis for a speech evaluation, I always have to find out how well a child is hearing. If a child is not hearing well, she is not likely to speak well or understand language well. Parents often report that a child has had recurrent middle ear infections. Sometimes the child has a lot of ear wax blocking the ability to hear sounds and parents are unaware of how poorly the child is hearing. Often, like Riley, the child is not complaining. Even a mild hearing loss can have large impact on a child's speech and language development.

I recommend that you take your child to an "Ear-Nose and Throat doctor" or "ENT" and a *pediatric audiologist.* Sometimes parents say, "Oh, his hearing was checked in the pediatrician's office and it's fine." The testing in the pediatrician's office is usually sufficient in other circumstances, but if your child has a speech or language concern, it is critical to get a thorough hearing evaluation. A pediatric audiologist can diagnose the hearing ability of infants and children of any age and any developmental status. If enough sounds are not coming into the brain, there will be changes in the auditory center of the brain, and if the auditory center is not stimulated with sound, it won't develop normally. As a result, speech and language will not develop normally.

There are different types of hearing loss.

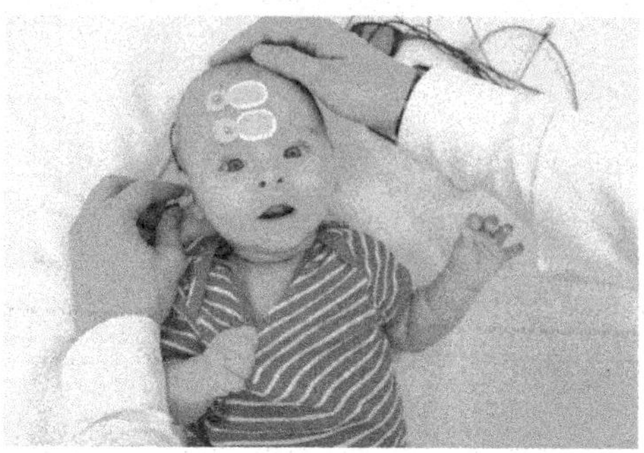

Congenital and acquired hearing loss

A hearing loss can be congenital, meaning present at birth, or it could be acquired. A common cause of an acquired hearing loss is fluid in the middle ears. A congenital hearing loss may mean, but does not necessarily mean, that hearing loss is an inherited trait. Ninety-five percent of children with a congenital hearing loss are born to parents who hear!

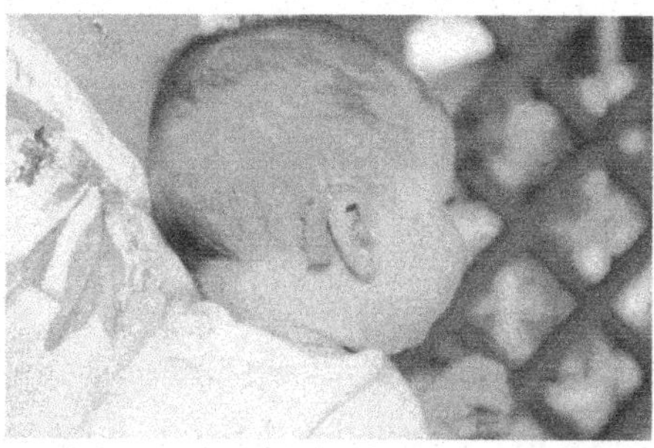

It is important that a child with a congenital hearing loss have hearing aids so that he will not miss important developmental milestones. Studies have shown that if a child with a congenital hearing loss is fitted appropriately with hearing aids before age 6 months, and wears the hearing aids for at least 10 hours per day, there will be no speech and language delay. For every 6 months that the child does not wear a hearing aid, there is a measurably *significant* delay. Infants fitted at 12 months have been shown to be one standard deviation below their peers in language development from typical peers; if fitted at 18 months, they are two standard deviations below their hearing peers and by age 2, they are likely to be 3 standard deviations below their hearing peers. Three standard deviations below means that the child is in the *bottom one percent* of all children in speech and language development – and this could be a child with normal cognitive abilities, just an inability to hear!

Conductive and Sensorineural Hearing Loss

A conductive hearing loss is lowered ability to hear sounds due to damage to the outer or middle ear, otitis media (commonly called a middle ear infection), a structural deformity, a cholesteatoma (a noncancerous skin growth in the middle ear) or foreign bodies in the ear. It means that not enough sound is sent to the brain.

By contrast, a person may have enough sound received by the outer and middle ear, but the sound is not being transmitted to the brain by the inner ear. This is a sensorineural hearing loss and is caused by hair cell damage in the cochlea, damage to the eighth cranial nerve or auditory neuropathy spectrum disorder (ANSD) – a problem in the transmission of the signal. ANSD may not be detected during the newborn screening but becomes apparent later in the first year of life when the child doesn't seem to react to sounds. Sensorineural hearing loss could be congenital, genetic or caused by a fever or viral infection.

A child could also be diagnosed with a mixed hearing loss, meaning both conductive and sensorineural. So, when we say a child has a "hearing loss," it could mean a loss within any part of this elaborate system – outer ear (rarely), middle ear, inner ear, the auditory pathway to the brain or the auditory center of the brain.

Sounds come in a range of frequencies. Sounds with high frequencies we perceive as high-pitched sounds and sounds with lower frequencies we perceive as low pitch. Different speech sounds in English have different frequencies. For example, the "m" sound is about 250 Hz, but an "s" sound is about 4000Hz. The audiologist will measure how well your child hears the different frequencies. A child with a high frequency hearing loss, for example, may clearly hear words like "Mom" but may not clearly hear words like "sister." If the child is missing certain frequencies, he or she is missing parts of speech!

Measuring Hearing Loss

The audiologist will measure how loudly the sound must be presented for the child to hear it. For example, if it is described as a "50 decibel hearing loss," this means that sounds must be presented at 50db or higher for the child to hear it. The audiologist will describe the hearing loss on a scale from mild to severe.

If a child has a 50-decibel hearing loss, she is missing most normal conversation. If a child hears less than 70% of sounds, her hearing would be considered "poor."

Auditory Processing Disorders

Besides testing how well your child can hear, audiologists can test how well your child processes sounds. If a child has an auditory processing disorder, the ears are working but the path from the ears to the brain jumbles the message and the child can't make sense of the sounds. Children must be school-aged to be tested for auditory processing difficulties.

Some children are diagnosed with an auditory information disorder. The ears are working, but the child is too distracted to tune into the auditory information.

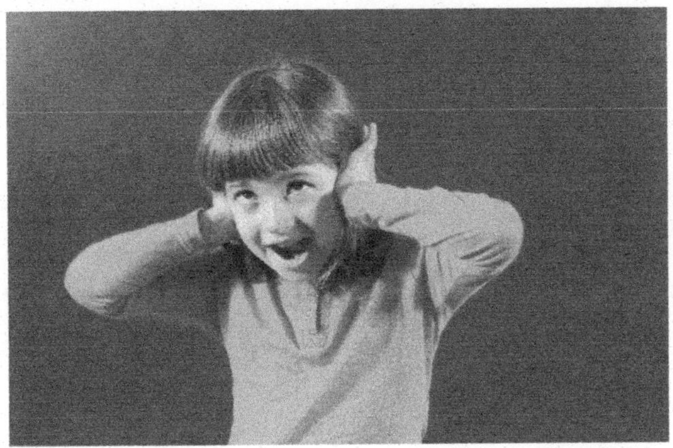

Sound Sensitivity

And finally, some children are diagnosed with sound sensitivity. The ears are working, but the child is unusually sensitive to normal sounds. For these children, the sounds of buzzing fluorescent lights in the classroom are so distracting, they can't concentrate on anything else! Having a child with sound sensitivity does not mean that your child has autism, but many children diagnosed with autism also have sound sensitivities.

How children learn to hear

Children learn to perceive sound and filter sound in a developmental order. For example, a very young baby will startle from any sound—rustling paper, or a spoon dropping. As the baby grows, he learns to recognize certain sounds and not startle when the sound is not novel or alarming. He also learns to filters sounds into *foreground* and *background*. If you, an adult, are working and a noisy garbage truck comes down the street, you will pay no heed to the background noise of the garbage truck, because it is a familiar sound that you have learned to put into the background of your auditory field. The same noise will make a three-year-old will run to the window, because he has not yet learned to filter the garbage truck sounds into the background.

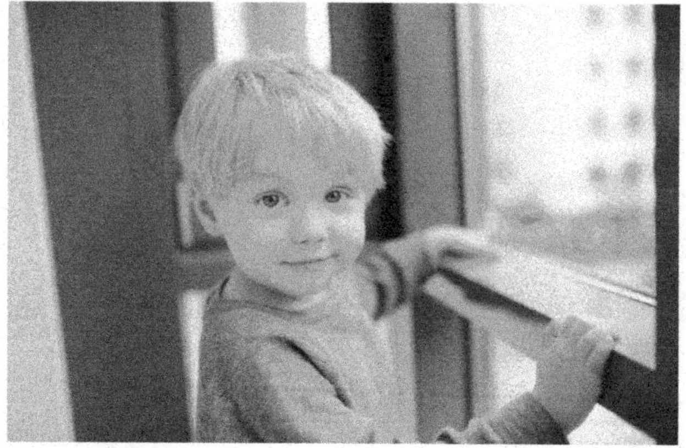

A child learns to recognize and reproduce sounds in his own language. Babies can babble many sounds that would be familiar to speakers of different languages, but as the baby grows, he perceives the sounds in his own language and eventually only babbles those sounds.

Children learn to perceive speech sounds in a developmental order. There are certain periods of time in which a child is developmentally ready to perceive a set of speech sounds. If the child has a middle ear infection during that time and never heard those sounds well enough, the child may have difficulty producing those sounds later on and will need speech therapy to learn those sounds. As a speech pathologist, I notice that the child often distorts sounds not learned at the correct developmental time.

From the moment a baby is born, she listens to the language around her. A newborn baby can perceive all the speech sounds of all the languages of the world, but at about six months, she gradually notices which speech sounds she hears most often. Her perception of speech sounds narrows and she loses the ability to recognize the difference in sounds that are not part of the language she hears around her. First, she recognizes vowel sounds in her own language and by 12 months, recognizes consonant sounds in her native language. She also begins to perceive how these sounds are assembled into words in her native language. For example, a made-up word like "grinch" has an acceptable combination of sounds in the English language, whereas "nigrch" does not.

As the baby continues to filter sounds into native and non-native, she gradually loses her ability to discern differences in sounds in non-native languages.

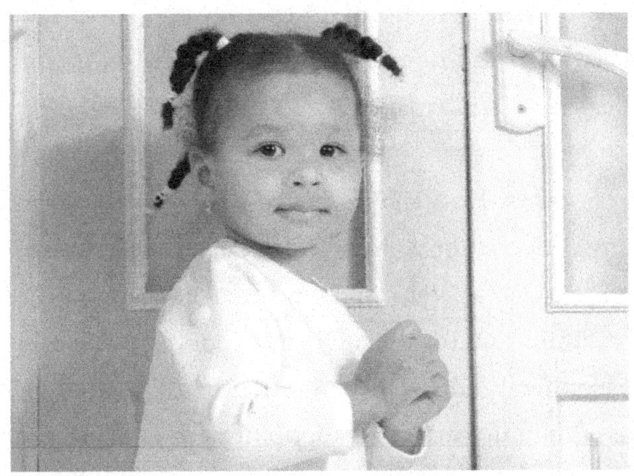

This is Jordan. Jordan is a 3-year-old girl who had frequent ear infections for much of her infancy. She had "tubes" inserted in her ears just two months ago. Her hearing has improved but it is still difficult to understand Jordan's speech because she distorts sounds in words. She scored in the 2nd percentile on a test of receptive language. Jordan is diagnosed with a speech/language delay due to hearing loss.

There are significant consequences for children who don't hear well

A child must hear well enough to learn. If a child is not hearing well, she will not learn speech and language well. She may have difficulty learning to read. It has been estimated that a child must first have 20,000 hours of listening to sounds to learn to read. If we don't know how your child is hearing, we can't diagnose a speech or language disorder with any certainty. Your child must hear well in order to learn to speak.

A speech delay is not just associated with children who are *severely* hearing impaired. About a quarter of kids will have an ear infection by the age of one, and 60% by age four. A child with chronic ear infections has periods of time when he is not hearing. When he is not hearing, he is not learning speech and language like a normal child. He may be missing development sound perception for that age and may need to be *taught* those sounds later. In addition, a child with an overabundance of ear wax may not be hearing as a normal child.

Checklist for Parents: How's My Child Doing?

If you have any concern about your child's speech or language, please find a pediatric audiologist in your area and make an appointment for your child. It is very important to rule out hearing loss as a cause for a speech or language developmental delay. If your child has a hearing loss, this must be taken care of first. If you have an appointment to bring your child for a speech/language evaluation, please also bring your child's medical record so you can accurately describe how many ear infections your child has had, and whether or not there were "tubes" put in and when.

5

LANGUAGE DISORDERS

What is a language disorder?

As we discussed, speech is talking. Language is a method of communication that consists of words used in a structured way. Language can be conveyed by speech, signing, writing or gesture. A child may not be speaking well because he has a language disorder. A person with a cognitive impairment often has a language disorder. However, a person with a language disorder does not necessarily have a cognitive impairment.

A child with a *receptive* language disorder has difficulty understanding what is said. A toddler with a receptive language disorder may struggle to follow simple directions, such as "Go into the bedroom and get your teddy bear."

A child with an *expressive* language disorder has trouble putting phrases and sentences together that are grammatical and convey the intended meaning. For example, a typical two-year-old will use two-and-three-word phrases to convey an idea, such as saying *Puppy sick!* or *I need help!* A child with an expressive language disorder may mimic vomiting sounds to indicate that the puppy is sick, but does not yet know how to put the words together to say puppy sick. He may cry or whine or bang his toy when he needs help, but he cannot put the words together to say "I need help."

What is the difference between a language disorder and a speech disorder?

A language disorder is different from a speech disorder. In a speech disorder, the child has difficulty physically forming words so that someone can understand what he is saying. A child with a speech disorder may be able to say "I want milk" but you may not be able to understand what he is saying because he cannot say the speech sounds clearly. A child with a language disorder doesn't know how to assemble words in the correct order to communicate to his parent: "I want milk." A child with a speech disorder may say "I'm donna doe to Tatie's house," In this sentence, the language is structured in an acceptable way, but the child cannot produce a /g/ or /k/ sound. This child may have a *speech disorder* but not a *language disorder*. A child with a language disorder may say *Kate-Kate house* for the same idea.

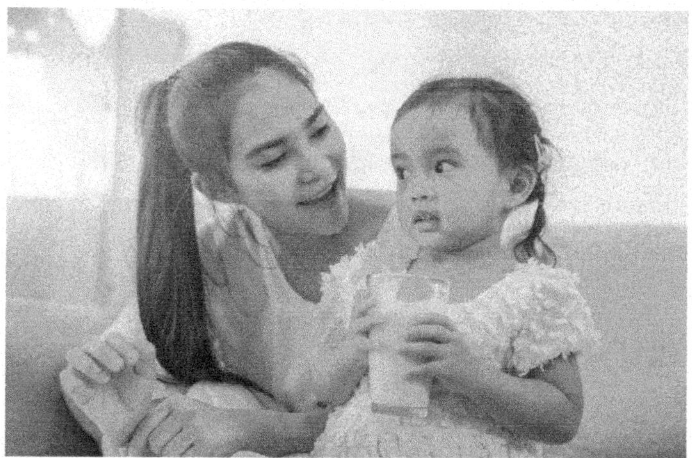

Some children have just an expressive language disorder, some have both a receptive and expressive language disorder. And, of course, a child may have a speech disorder *with* a language disorder or may have a speech disorder *without* a language disorder. A good speech pathologist can diagnose just where the child is struggling.

How can I tell if my child has a language disorder?

A toddler with a receptive language disorder often has difficulty understanding what is said to him. He may not understand the meaning of key words, such as "put that *under the chair*" or "The teacher gave the present to *him*." A young child with an expressive language disorder generally has a lower overall vocabulary than most children his age. He may struggle to put sentences together and speak grammatically. He may struggle to explain what he saw or what happened to him.

By age four or five, a child should be able to tell you something about a movie he watched. If he enjoys repeating lines from movies, but has difficulty telling what the movie is about, he may have difficulty using language. The child may mimic sounds in the movie, such as "*swwwwish!*" or may repeat a favorite line, such as "I can't see why not!" or may re-enact an action scene, but cannot say, "Spiderman fights the bad guy!"

What causes a language disorder?

We may not know for sure. One possible reason is that language disorders run in the family. Some genes have been identified as related to speech and language disorders. Being born prematurely, with a low birth weight or with hearing loss may result in a language disorder. If a child has a more comprehensive diagnosis, such as autism, a syndrome, a cognitive impairment or a brain injury, a language disorder may be part of the more comprehensive diagnosis. For example, many children with autism are *very* late talkers and continue to have difficulty with language, particularly *pragmatic* or *social* language for a lifetime. Children with Williams Syndrome, as part of the syndrome, speak fluently but superficially.

How prevalent are language disorders?

They appear to affect 6-15% of children and more boys than girls.

How is a language disorder diagnosed?

There are a variety of normed, standardized language assessments used by speech-language pathologists to determine if a child's ability to understand and use language is age-appropriate. A child who is under three years old and barely verbal is usually assessed with a developmental test. Once the child is over three, a speech pathologist will use a standardized language assessment for diagnosis.

There is quite a bit of variability in language development in one-year-olds. Once your child turns two, however, if he is saying fewer than fifty words and does not make any unique two-word combinations such as *"Daddy home!" or "puppy sick,"* your child would be considered a "late talker." Most late talkers have labelling words, such as *puppy, car, keys, Mama, ball* but few or no action words, such as *wash, cut, eat, jump.* I consider age two to be the "line in the sand." If your child does not have a vocabulary of fifty words and is not combining words together by the second birthday, it is time to seek help. It will only benefit your child.

My child struggles to answer questions. Is this a language disorder?

If your child cannot answer age-appropriate questions, he may not understand the words of the question and may have a language disorder.

Some children almost always answer questions with the last words of the question. If you ask, "Do you want a cookie?" the child will answer "cookie" or "want a cookie." If you ask, "Did you go to Grandma's house?" the child answers "Grandma's house." This indicates that the child does not understand the question and is struggling with language.

We often see children in our office who use *associated* words to describe things or answer questions, and this indicates a language disorder. Here is an example from a little boy in our office:

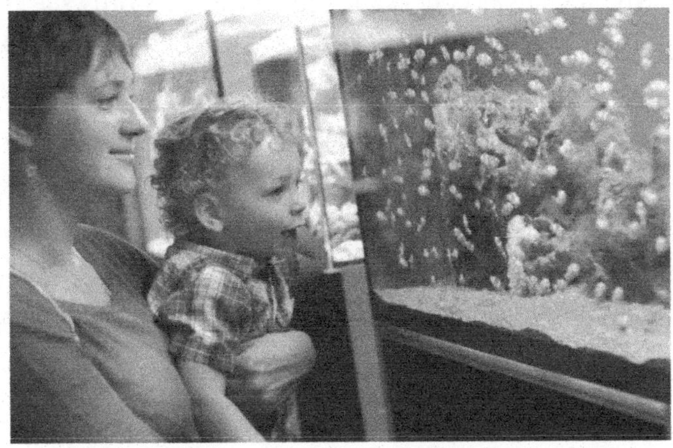

This is Patrick. His parents are concerned that he has difficulty understanding questions. He repeats the last word or words of every question. For example, if they ask him "Do you want a cookie?" Patrick will answer "cookie". He observes routines, and helps prepare his bath every night by turning on the light and getting the bubbles. His parents haven't heard him speak in sentences; he gives one-word answers most of the time. Patrick often uses words associated with a previous experience to describe something. For example, when he entered our speech therapy clinic, he approached the fish tank and saw a fish similar to a fish he saw recently at the local taco restaurant. Patrick pointed to the fish and said to his parents, "Taco! Taco!"

This little boy repeats words he heard when he had a similar experience. Using an associated word to describe an activity or answering a question with the last word or words of the question is often observed in children with autism. It indicates that he does not understand language well enough to communicate his experiences with appropriate words.

Echolalia indicates a language disorder.

A child may echo phrases that she hears. My 2-year-old granddaughter heard her father say, "I don't know if we can make it." She repeated over and over to herself, "make it…. make it." This is called verbal play and it is normal. The child is just practicing an interesting word or phrase. However, if the child *usually* answers questions with the last words she heard or a repeated phrase, that may mean that the child does not understand the question. For example, if you ask your child, "Do you want juice?" and she answers "want juice" and then you ask her "Did you find those shoes?" and she answers "find those shoes," this is echolalia. She is not answering the question, she is repeating the last words she heard. A child may have heard a character in a movie say, "I can't see why not!" If she often answers questions with that phrase, she may be exhibiting *delayed echolalia*. She heard the phrase before and uses it when she perceives she needs to produce an answer. Echolalia, when used frequently and without understanding, can be an early sign of autism.

We do not speak English at home. Will this cause a language disorder in my child?

No! Children all over the world learn to speak other languages. Speak to your child in the language that you know best. A typical child will benefit tremendously from being fluent in both languages. If your child struggles with *both* languages, he may have a language disorder.

What about twins? Do twins develop language later than singles?

Late talking is more common in twins. It may be because statistically, more twins are premature or low birthweight babies. It may be because "twin language," which the twins speak to each other and may not use words we understand. An interesting study showed that twins used fewer words and simpler language when speaking to each other.

Will a language disorder affect my child's ability to learn to read?

Many studies have found that children with speech sound disorders and language disorders are at increased risk for reading disorder. Children diagnosed with language disorders with no known cause as preschoolers are at least four times more likely to have reading disabilities than other children. A large-scale study of kindergarteners followed for several years showed that the majority of those with language disorders continued to exhibit language and/or academic difficulties through adolescence.

For children with a mild intellectual disability, a language disorder may be subtle, including difficulty with abstract language or social communication.

What is narrative language and why is it important for a child to use narratives?

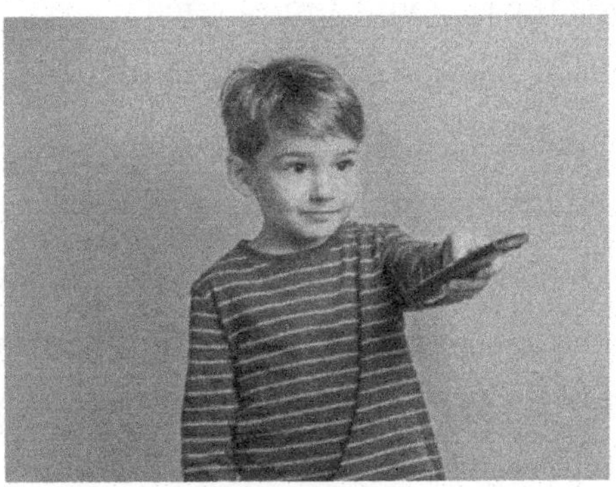

This is Brian. Brian loves to watch movies. He likes to reenact his favorite action sequences, but it seems like he doesn't really understand the movie. He also struggles with reading comprehension. Could this be related?"

Brian may be struggling with narrative language. Children and adults use narrative language to create stories and describe what is happening in their daily lives. Although you may think "telling narratives" is "creative writing," oral narratives are actually the structure underlying our communication with others.

Think of the structure underlying a simple story you might tell a friend. "I had ants on my kitchen countertop, so I put out ant traps. I still had ants! Then I heard that honey and baking powder would trap the ants, so I did that. I still had ants! Finally, I just called the exterminator and now there are no ants on my countertop. I feel better cooking dinner now." In this short narrative, you identify what you want (a sanitary countertop) and what your problem is (ants). You then tell your friend the steps you took to solve the problem. There is a resolution and an emotional reaction to the events. This is a narrative structure. If you leave out any elements, your friend will not understand your story.

By kindergarten, a child should inherently understand narrative structure. He might be able to tell you what happened to him, such as "Today we had a race. I wanted to win! I started running really fast, but then my shoelace untied. When I stopped to tie my shoelace, another kid ran past me and won the ribbon! I almost cried!"

A child who does not understand narrative structure will not be able to tell you what happened to him and will also have difficulty understanding written stories and television programs that tell a story.

Difficulty with language comprehension is sometimes mistaken for a reading comprehension difficulty. Some children can hide a language disorder until they begin to fall behind in reading comprehension. When they are tested in school, it is discovered that the child can read, but can't understand the language that underlies the reading.

Checklist for Parents: How's My Child Doing?

I'm sure you videotape your child doing cute things regularly! If your child is shy or you're concerned that she may not speak as usual during an evaluation, please take a 30 second video of your child speaking at home and bring it to the evaluation with you.

When to bring your child to a developmental pediatrician

As speech-language pathologists, we measure a child's language abilities. Often, children do not display joint attention and communicative intent or do not have age-appropriate language skills because there is an underlying condition, such as ADHD or autism or a syndrome. Speech-language pathologists do not generally diagnose these conditions, but refer you to a developmental pediatrician if a condition is suspected. During my evaluation, I look for signs of autism and if there are several, I will refer the parent for further testing with a developmental pediatrician. During your child's evaluation, you can ask if a referral to a developmental pediatrician is warranted.

PART II

Speech

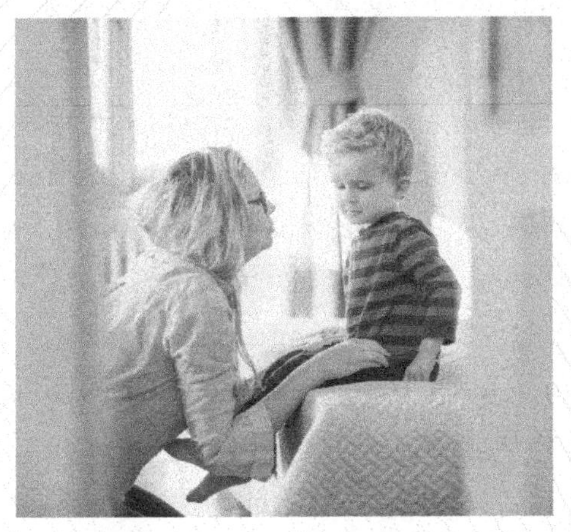

Your child is trying to communicate with you. Perhaps *you* know what he's trying to say, but the words are not clear yet. When your child speaks to Grandma or the clerk in the store or to other children, you often have to interpret for your child.

Maybe your child uses mostly gestures and only simple words. Maybe your child mixes up speech sounds and it is hard to understand what she is saying. Maybe your child lisps.

There are many different reasons why a child may not speak clearly. In this section, I will tell you how most children develop the ability to speak and then I will tell you what types of speech difficulties we see every day in our clinic. This should help you to narrow down just *why* your child is struggling.

6

HOW DO CHILDREN LEARN TO SPEAK?

Speech is talking – using the muscles of the tongue, lips, jaw and vocal tract in a very precise and coordinated way to produce the sounds that make up language. If your child has a speech sound disorder, she has difficulty using the mechanics of speaking for clear articulation, voice and fluency. We have covered language development; here we are discussing speech development.

Speech is the most complex motor activity that any person acquires. When we talk or sing, we release controlled puffs of air from our lungs through our larynx and vocal cords. By shaping that air with the throat, tongue and lips, we produce a specific sound – like an ah or dada. But sounds cannot be formed randomly. They must be precisely sequenced to form words, produced with the right pitch for intonation and with enough air to speak an entire sentence. It requires an enormous amount of fine motor control.

Is there a difference between "typical" development and "normal" development?

Yes. Researchers have spent years trying to figure out at what age the majority of children understand or say different things. Hence, when we say "the typical child puts two words together by the second birthday," it means researchers assembled the age at which 1,000 children put two words together, put it into a bell-curve statistical analysis and determined that 24 months was "average." Your child may be on either side of the Bell

Curve, either putting two words together much earlier or much later and still be "normal." It is much like saying "the average American child weighs 27 pounds at age 24 months." You could still have a healthy child who weighs more or less than the average. But if your child weighs more or less than average *for a reason*, such as an underlying anomaly or illness, your child's weight may not be *normal*. And, of course, the further your child is from *average*, the greater the chance that his speech development may not be *normal*.

Is My Child's Speech Normal?

What is "normal" in a child of one age may not be "normal" in an older child. For example, many two-year-olds will say "I donna doe" for *I'm gonna go.* This is appropriate for a two-year old, but by age three, most children perceive and produce the /g/ sound.

There are some things that are not "normal" at any age. If your child deletes the *first sound* in most words, this is not normal. If your child has an open mouth posture, with his tongue protruding and difficulty containing saliva, this is not normal. If your child makes an "uh" sound in the middle of words, such as chuh-eese for *cheese,* this is not normal. These are things that need to be addressed by a Speech pathologist and corrected so that your child can continue to make progress with his speech.

What is a speech sound disorder?

A child who cannot speak clearly for his age is said to have a speech sound disorder. This is not a cognitive disorder; the child just has difficulty speaking clearly.

How common are speech sound disorders in children?

Speech sound disorders are quite common in preschoolers and are less common as children get older. More boys than girls have speech sound disorders. Estimates vary, but about 15% of 3-year-olds have some sort of speech sound disorder. By age 6, only 4% of children have a speech sound disorder. Keep in mind that many preschoolers have received speech therapy and that significantly reduces speech sound disorders.

Although many children with speech sound disorders as preschoolers will progress into the normal range by the time they begin kindergarten, speech sound disorders are associated with an increased risk of reading, writing, or spelling disorders.

It is important to know that having a speech sound disorder does not mean that the child has a cognitive deficit. Many normal and very bright children have speech sound disorders. I often meet parents who are reluctant to enroll their child in speech therapy because they don't want their child identified as impaired. I tell them that if their child needed glasses to see well, they would get him glasses so that he does not *become* impaired. A child with a speech sound disorder needs a boost from speech therapy so that he can go on to lead his best life.

Can a child have more than one speech sound disorder concurrently?

Yes, it is possible.

What are the consequences of not addressing my child's speech sound disorder?

A child needs to have intelligible speech by age 5 ½ or he is likely to have difficulty in school. He may struggle with spelling, writing and being understood.

Parents can be afraid that their child's speech difficulty will be noticed by peers. In my experience, classmates don't notice the speech disorders of their peers in the very early years of school – kindergarten and first grade. Children of this age don't mind "going to speech" in either school or private therapy. By third grade, classmates notice which children in their class don't speak clearly and it is no longer fun to be pulled out for speech in school.

How are speech sound disorders treated?

One size does not fit all! Speech sounds disorders are remedied by treating the cause of the disorder and is tailored to fit your child's needs. A child with a muscle-based disorder will be treated with muscle-strengthening exercises. A child with a phonological disorder will be taught to listen to sounds and reproduce individual sounds. A child with apraxia will start reproducing easier word "shapes" and gradually add motor complexity to words.

It is the job of the speech-language pathologist to determine the most appropriate methods to use with each child. Truth be told, speech pathology is an art as well as a science. A good clinician often uses some techniques from this program and some from that program and some from our experience working with children with similar struggles in the past.

Is normal speech development different for an internationally adopted child?

Deborah Hwa-Froelich is a researcher who studied speech development with internationally adopted children. She found that children can acquire their new language within two to three years after adoption. However, the child's care before being adopted may affect his ability to acquire his adoptive language. Did he come from a nurturing environment? Did he have adequate nutrition? Did he have access to medical care? If not, his language development may be delayed for these reasons. Or, these reasons could affect his ability to develop attention, and that would affect his language development once adopted.

* * *

Parents consider baby's first word to be a milestone, and indeed it is. Consider what abilities your child must develop *before* producing his first recognizable word - your baby must have:

* normal hearing ability

* the ability to coordinate breathing so that a word is said on the exhale

* normal mouth structures; if the baby's palate is not fused properly or the frenum under the tongue is too tight or the lips do not meet properly, there will not be clear speech

* sufficient muscle strength to move the mouth, jaw, tongue and lips to form the sound

* the ability to perceive and imitate the correct sound; this is called phonological awareness. The baby's brain must perceive the difference between a /d/ and an /m/ sound to correctly say *Dada* and *Mama*.

* the ability to coordinate a sequence of motor movements in the correct order.

If your child struggles in any one of these areas, it will be evident in unclear speech.

A speech delay may be the first indication that the child is struggling with one of these sub-skills. In the following chapter, I will discuss what is considered typical speech development. In subsequent chapters, I will discuss the various reasons why your child may be struggling with speech sounds.

7

TYPICAL CHILD SPEECH DEVELOPMENT & MILESTONES

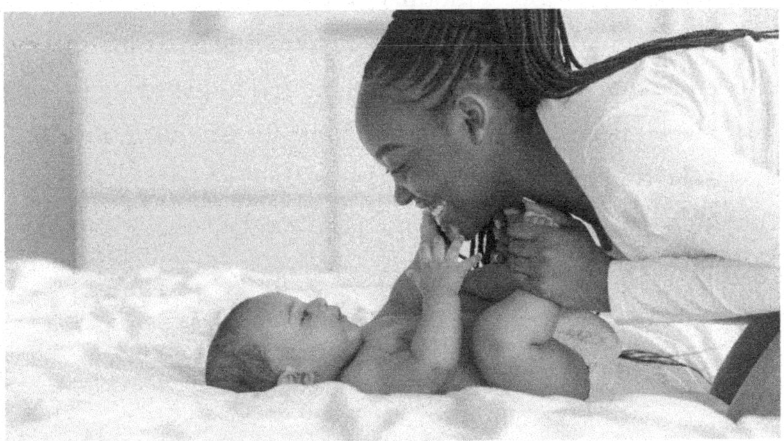

How does speech develop during the first year?

The first sounds a baby makes are reflexive. That means he doesn't need to *learn* to make the sound. A newborn baby cries. Crying is inhalation followed by vocalization. The infant reflexively changes the pitch and intensity of his cry in response to the situation. Reflexive sounds also include grunts when pooping, burps, hiccups and coughing. As a newborn, he cannot yet make vowel and consonant sounds because his tongue is now very large in his mouth. He needs a large tongue to form a seal onto his mother's nipple and nurse. Any speech sounds he produces now are with a closed or nearly closed mouth, so they are nasal sounds, like /m/.

By months two to four, most typically-developing infants begin to coo. Cooing is making vowel sounds, like *a-a-a-a*. And, the baby is starting to pay attention to sounds. If you gaze into your baby's face and imitate his sounds, he will respond to you and continue to make those sounds. By the fourth month, many babies will start to laugh!

Anywhere from 3 ½ months until 8 months, the baby begins *vocal play*. He is gaining more control of his body and can now vocalize *intentionally*. He is also learning to change the loudness and pitch of his vocalizations.

Babbling begins at 6 ½ months to 8 months. The first kind of babbling is a string of consonant plus vowel sounds such as ma-ma-ma-ma or bee-bee-bee-bee. The consonant is the same and the string is said over and over. Babbling is an important milestone for parents to note because the baby is developing motor control. Some children later diagnosed with speech motor control difficulty did not babble as babies.

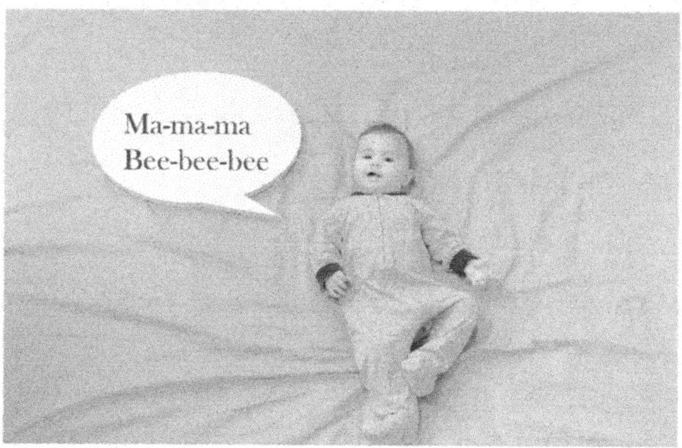

Beginning at about 10-14 months, the baby learns to vary the sounds he babbles. Now instead of bee-bee-bee-bee, he is saying bee-dee-bee-dee-bee-dee or da-dee-da-dee-da-dee. Your baby is able to do this now because his vocal tract is lengthening, his facial bones are growing downward and forward and he has increased control of his tongue. If your baby is *not* babbling at this point, it is important to bring him to a pediatric audiologist and have his hearing checked.

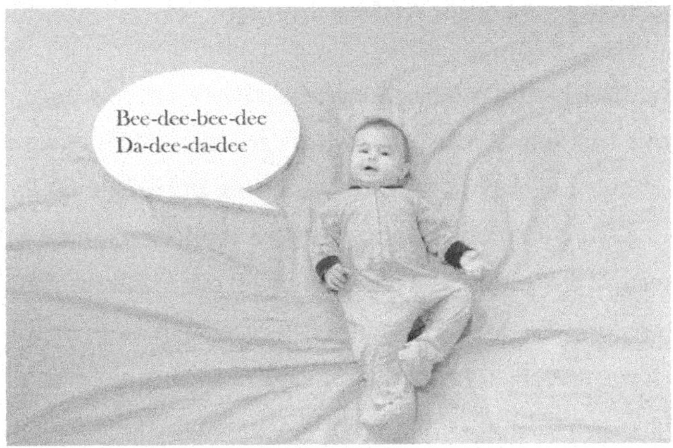

After this, your child begins to speak in *jargon*. *Jargon* means that the baby imitates the speech sounds and intonation of his native language without saying any actual words. This is a very cute stage in which the baby seems to be saying something to you very earnestly, but there are no actual words. From a baby's jargon, you can tell if the child is being raised in an English-speaking household or a French-speaking household or a Japanese-speaking household. The baby now perceives the *rhythm* of his native language.

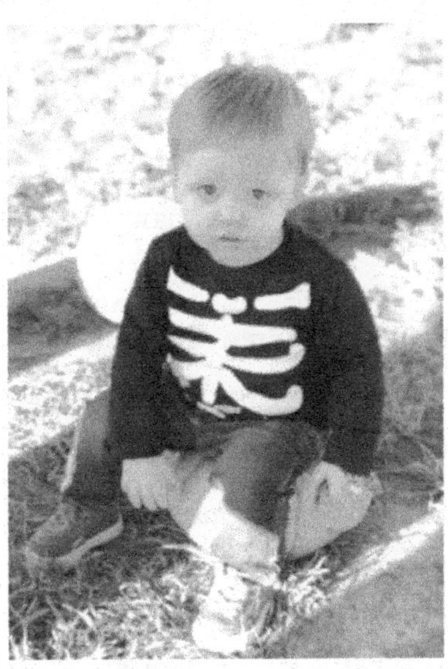

What should my one-year-old be saying?

At about the first birthday, the moment arrives that you have been waiting for: baby's first word! Most first words are two-syllable words with the same consonant-vowel pair repeated, such as *mama* or *dada*, and then *Nana or Papa, baba* for a bottle, *nana* for a banana. Consonant-vowel combinations are the easiest for the child to say, so you will notice many consonant-vowel combinations. Popular words are farm animals sounds: *moo, baa, neigh.* Your baby will probably repeat the sound, such as *moo-moo* or *neigh-neigh.* Animal sounds that are not consonant-vowel may be said as consonant-vowel, such as *woo* instead of *woof, pee* instead of *peep.* This is normal. My one-year-old grandson's favorite word is "car." We think of the word as a consonant-vowel-consonant but the sounds are really just /k/ and /ah/ - consonant vowel, which is age-appropriate.

Most babies don't yet have the physical ability to put a consonant on the end of a word yet. Consonants are formed with the lips, tongue and teeth. Vowels are formed by adjusting the shape of the opening of the vocal tract; it takes more coordination to add consonant to the end of the word than the baby has right now.

When children begin saying early words, they often use their entire tongue and jaw to say it. For example, your child may say *dada* by bringing her tongue to her palate with her jaw. As she gets older, she will learn to move her tongue independently of her jaw and will say *dada* by simply elevating her tongue.

This is the age at which children also first start to greet people, saying *hi, bye-bye* .and *nie-nie* (for night-night). Is it any wonder that these are consonant-vowel words?

The next stage for the typical one-year-old is to start to change the consonants or vowels in consonant-vowel words. So, *mama* becomes *mommy* and words like *baby* and *nanny* start to appear. After this, the baby is able to add a final consonant to words. Most first words have the same consonant repeated, like *pop,* but then the baby learns to change the final consonant to say words like *hot, hat* and *sock.*

Your baby is now communicating with you using single words. These single words can be used for different purposes, and sometimes it's not clear just what the child means. My little granddaughter, Cora, liked to find the cat when she came to our house, even though she was a little bit afraid of him. When she found the cat, she would stand a few feet away from him and point her finger and say, "Nice!" Of course, we did not know if she was trying to tell us that *the cat is nice* or if she was congratulating herself for finding the cat, or if she was afraid he may come towards her and wanted to remind him: *Be nice!*

Even when real words are emerging, your child will continue to babble and use jargon. Think of babbling and jargon as vocal play. You may hear your child talking to herself in her crib, mixing a steady stream of jargon with a few clear words.

At about age 19 months, in addition to words that identify people and objects, your child will start using action words.It is now possible to put two words together in a subject-action sentence: *Doggy sit! Daddy go.* Many children will put request *more,* such as *more* juice at 20 months and say give *me* at 22 months.

Before your child produces a real word, he may say a quasi-word, which is a child-invented word that is used consistently, but does not sound like the real word. He may say *gee* for his stuffed bunny. Although the family knows that *gee* is the bunny, the word does not sound anything like *bunny,* so it is a quasi-word.

A real word is said *consistently,* meaning that he always says this word for this thing; *independently,* meaning that he can say the word without coaching and *intentionally,* meaning he is trying to communicate with the word.

What should my two-year-old be saying?

By the second birthday, the words your child says have changed. Instead of everything being consonant-vowel-consonant-vowel, such as *woo-woo* for the dog, the child can now put consonants at the end of words, and say "dog." Some children may reverse /d/ with /g/ and call him a "gog" or a "dod" but there is a final consonant there!

Your child may substitute some sounds for others. He may call the cat a "tat," or say "wittle" for *little* or "I donna doe" for "I'm gonna go." This is age-appropriate because your child is just learning to produce speech sounds.

By the second birthday, the typical child has a vocabulary of about 260 words and can put two words together, such as "Daddy home" or "puppy sick." A favorite word is "no!" You may hear, "No night night!" The important thing is that the child is communicating by uniquely putting two words together. So, "thank you" or "bye-bye" are two-word phrases, but they are memorized phrases so this is not considered putting two words together.

Now his vocabulary will expand rapidly. He will talk about things that are not in the room with him. He will begin to use words like *in, on, under.* He will start to understand opposites, like *stop-go, big-little* and *up-down.* His speech should be clear enough that people who know him, including grandparents, can understand what he is saying.

Most children have a vocabulary of about 50 words before they put two words together. A child who says fewer than 50 words and is not yet putting two words together at 24 months would be called a "late talker."

Does late talking at age 2 mean that your child has a disability?

Not necessarily. There are children who are late bloomers and will catch up on their own. If your child was born prematurely, use the date he was due to be born and measure how much he is speaking by that date.

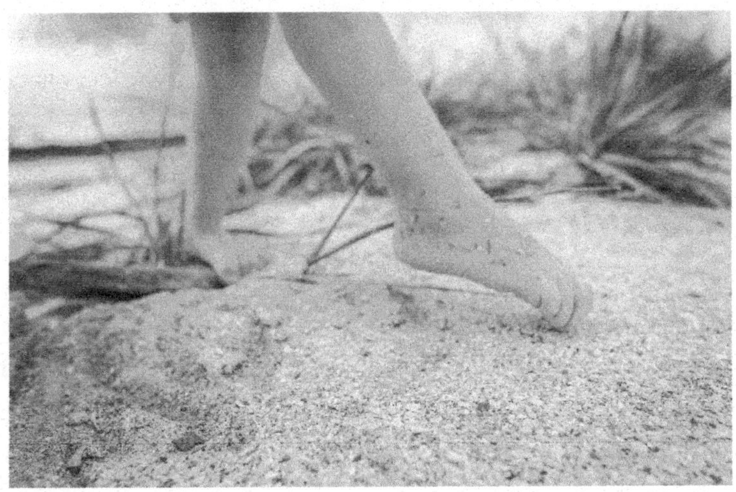

I would consider the second birthday to be the line in the sand:

If your child does not have a vocabulary of 50 words and is not combining two words together or cannot be understood, it is time for a speech evaluation.

What should my 3-year-old be saying?

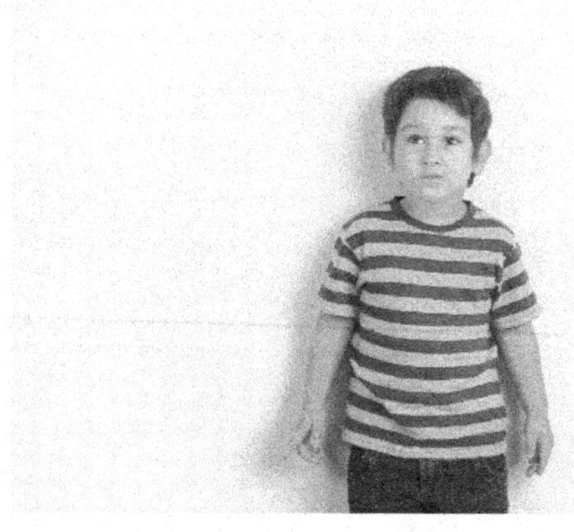

Three-year-olds are a delight! They are curious about the world around them and sometimes very funny in the way they perceive everyday experiences. My little granddaughter Caileigh did not have any brothers when she watched her baby cousin, Jack, have his diaper changed. She was shocked and said, "Oh my! Jack has a tail!"

The typical 3-year-old can name all extended family members, including aunts and uncles and cousins. He can identify shapes and colors. If you ask him what happened during the day, he can tell you. He can answer questions about who, what and where. He uses pronouns, such as *I pet the cat and he pet the cat, too. We both pet the cat!* By this point, most people can understand what he is saying.

What should my 4-year-old be saying?

By age 4, most children share their interpretation of the world with you. The child can tell you a short story, and use words like *first this happened and then--the last thing was--*or *yesterday I wanted this but today--and tomorrow.* By now, the typical child is socially aware and can fill in a conversation to keep it going. He also knows enough to speak differently to different people, using polite words to the teacher and keep his voice quieter indoors than outdoors.

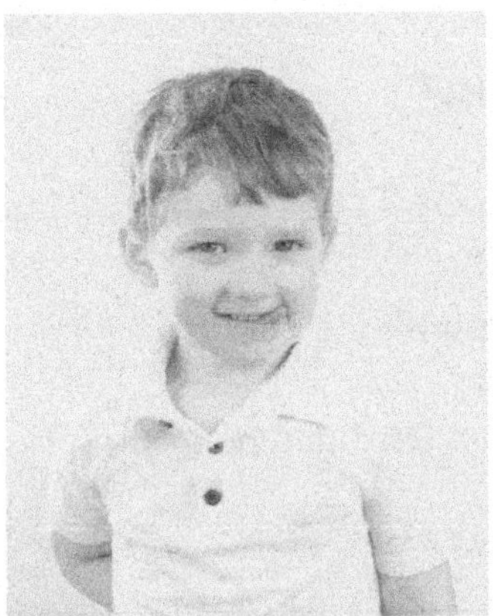

By the fourth birthday, the typical child speaks almost like an adult. He may not have mastered some speech sounds, and may still substitute /w/ for /r/, such as saying *wed wabbit* for "red rabbit" and substitute /f/ for /th/ and say *baf.* But other sounds should be mastered at this age.

At what age should my child speak clearly?

* *The typical 2-year-old child should be understandable to her parents and perhaps her grandparents. The typical 3-year-old child should be understandable to her grandparents and to adults who know her. The typical 4-year-old should be understandable to people who don't know her. Unless a child has a diagnosed disability, she should have clear speech by age 5½.*

All children should have *intelligible* speech by age 5 ½. "Intelligible" does not mean "intelligent;" it means clear speech. A perfectly *intelligent* child may not have *intelligible speech* for a variety of reasons.

If your child's speech is not *intelligible* by age 5 ½, he will struggle in school, usually with reading. It may be difficult for the child to associate letters with speech sounds and sequence sounds in reading words. This could be so exhausting to your child that she may not have enough energy left for reading fluency and reading comprehension.

How's My Child Doing?

NEWBORN TO 3 MONTHS

makes cooing sounds
smiles at people
has different cries for different needs

4 MONTHS TO 6 MONTHS

coos and babbles when playing alone or with you
makes consonant-vowel babbling sounds, such as *ba, pa, me*
giggles and laughs
makes sounds when happy or upset

7 TO 12 MONTHS

babbles a longer string of sounds; *me-me-me* or *ba-ba-ba-ba*
imitates some speech sounds
says one or two words around the first birthday

BY THE FIRST BIRTHDAY

Says one recognizable word with meaning, such as *Mama, Dada, baba.* If the baby is babbling *mama, mama, mama* but does not associate this sound with his mother, it would be considered babbling rather than a word.

12 TO 18 MONTHS

uses many new words
still uses jargon with some real words
babbles words with either a string of the same consonant-vowel syllable *(da-da-da)* or different consonant-vowel patterns *(da-di, pa-pi)*

18 TO 24 MONTHS

has a few recognizable words. The earliest words often have the same consonant and vowel repeated, such as *Dada, Mama, Baba, Papa, Nana, BeeBee*

WHAT ARE SOME SIGNS THAT I SHOULD BRING MY 2-YEAR-OLD FOR A SPEECH EVALUATION?

The child has fewer than 50 words in his vocabulary

The child is not combining words into unique phrases, such as *Daddy home!* or *Puppy sick!*

The child is labeling objects, but has no words for actions

The child appears to be struggling to speak

The child is exhibiting frustration at not being understood

WHAT ARE SOME SIGNS THAT I SHOULD BRING MY 3-YEAR-OLD FOR A SPEECH EVALUATION?

The child reduces words to simpler words, such as *neigh-neigh* for a horse

The child cannot produce consonant-vowel-consonant words, such as *cat, mouse, tub*

The child is not speaking in short sentences.

The child cannot produce many speech sounds yet.

The child cannot be understood by people outside the family.

The child appears to be struggling when speaking.

WHAT ARE SOME SIGNS THAT I SHOULD BRING MY 4-YEAR-OLD FOR A SPEECH EVALUATION?

The child has not developed all speech sounds.

The child does not speak clearly.

The child cannot tell you about what happened to him during the day.

The child is not speaking to other children or adults who visit.

The child is struggling to learn letter sounds in pre-school.

The child appears to be struggling when speaking.

WHAT ARE SOME SIGNS THAT I SHOULD BRING MY 5-YEAR-OLD FOR A SPEECH EVALUATION?

The child's speech is not clear to everyone.

The child substitutes or omits sounds from words.

The child cannot re-tell a story or tell you what a movie is about.

The child appears to struggle when speaking.

The child struggles with multi-syllable words.

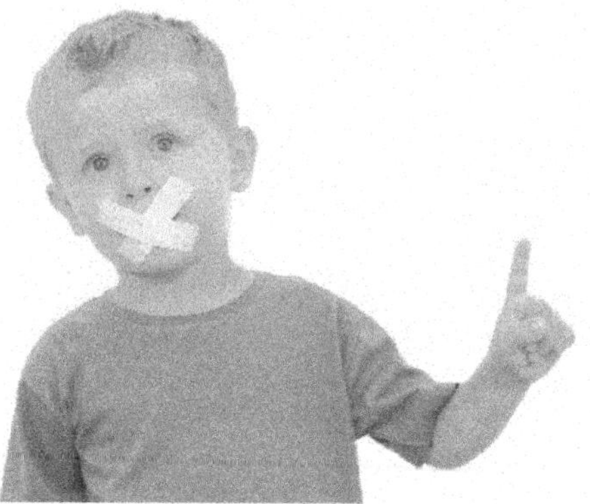

Why Doesn't My Child Speak Clearly?

Suppose your child wants to tell you, "I fell and got hurt." In order to say this clearly, your child must:

* have oral structures that allow for the movement necessary to accurately reproduce speech sounds

* control his breath and mouth movements necessary to produce the words

* use the correct muscles in the correct sequence with the correct timing to say the words

* correctly perceive and produce the speech sounds for the words

If one of these conditions are not met, your child will not have clear speech. A child with unclear speech is said to have a speech sound disorder.

The cause could be structural: the child cannot speak clearly because he has a cleft palate or a tongue tie or a tongue thrust. The child could have a phonological impairment, which means difficulty perceiving speech sounds correctly. He could have a motor speech impairment, which is difficulty actually producing the speech sounds. There are two types of motor impairments: dysarthria is difficulty with the muscle movement for speech sounds and apraxia is when the brain has difficulty planning the movement to make the speech sounds. Or, the child could have more than one reason for the speech sound impairment.

In this next section, I will tell you about different children who have come into my office with different types of speech sound disorders, and how each child was diagnosed.

8

STRUCTURAL ANOMALIES

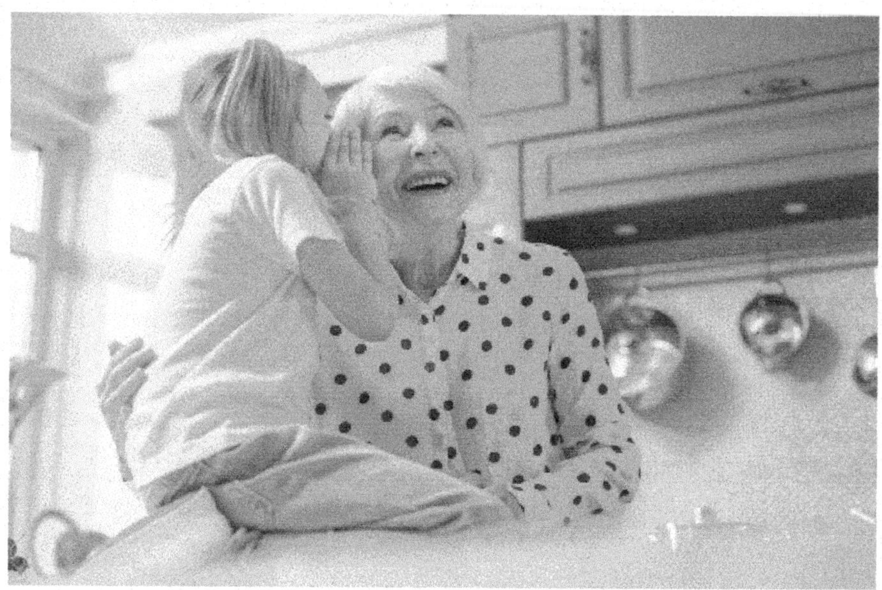

This is Reagan. Her mother, Heather, said this about Reagan:

My first pediatrician was not too concerned about Reagan, but I was. At fifteen months, Reagan wouldn't say more than the word "hi!" Everything was "hi, hi, hi!" Reagan was my second child and I don't know if I would have acted the same way if she was my first. I just knew that my older child spoke clearer and said lot more words at that age. When I pressed the pediatrician, he said we could inquire about an evaluation by early intervention, which we did, but Reagan didn't qualify. When she was about a year old, she started having a lot of ear infections. Once she got that first infection, it was one, after the next, after the next, after the next. She had tubes put in at seventeen months. At her two-year wellness visit, I said to the pediatrician, "She's still not saying more, she's had the tubes already, what's going on?" I had a gut feeling. I could tell that Reagan understood directions, but when she was repeating words back to me, it sounded like she was leaving off the ending sounds. My mom is a pre-school teacher and she really pushed me, saying, "It doesn't hurt to get a speech evaluation." I am a teacher, too, and I really believe that the sooner you address something, the sooner you're probably going to have success with any type of intervention. That's when I asked the doctor to write a referral for a speech evaluation.

Reagan qualified for speech therapy, but when we went back to the ENT to have her ears checked, we found out she had to have her tonsils out. That delayed speech therapy for a month, and then we were finally able to start up. Speech therapy definitely helped her to learn speech sounds! After the tonsils were out, her pre-school teacher called me and said, "Reagan is falling asleep in class." She was having a lot of sleep issues at home. The dentist noticed she was grinding her teeth. Her older sister, who shares a bunk bed with her, said, "Mom! I can't sleep at night because Reagan won't stop snoring!" I said, "Snoring! She's had her tonsils and adenoids out. What is going on?" I brought her back to the ENT doctor and he said, "Oh my God, she's got a full blockage on the left side of her nostril. She can't breathe at all! I have to do surgery on her. It's an ablation of the turbinate." Three weeks after that surgery, she had pink eye, even though we were in quarantine and hadn't left our house. The ENT said, "Look, you haven't left your house, I think we should consider allergy testing". I took her to the allergist and found out that she's highly allergic to dust mites and mold. That was causing all the blockages.

Reagan was struggling to speak because she had structural issue that affected her speech. Let me describe how structural issues may make it difficult for a child to speak clearly.

Some structural issues are congenital, meaning that the child is born with mouth structures that make it difficult to speak clearly. For example, if your child has a cleft palate, or a submucous cleft palate, air will escape into her nose unintentionally and her speech resonance will be impaired. If she has Down Syndrome, her eustachian tube will be lower and tilted and her tongue may be larger, making it more difficult to make accurate speech sounds. If she has velopharyngeal insufficiency, she cannot build up enough correct air pressure to make correct speech sounds. Children born with these issues may need a combination of surgery and speech therapy to achieve clear speech. However, a child may develop a structural issue as well, and it's important for you, as a parent, to make sure your child develops correctly. A common structural issue develops from chronic mouth breathing. Let me explain.

A newborn baby's mouth structures are different proportionally from an adult. The newborn's primary job is to *suckle* milk. Because suckling uses the tongue to pump the milk from the breast, the baby's tongue is proportionally bigger than an adult's and his larynx is higher. As the child grows and begins to sit up and eat table food, his tongue becomes proportionally smaller. Instead of the forward tongue that infants are so fond of sticking out, the tongue gradually sits behind the teeth. Ideally, your toddler will be resting his tongue on the roof of his mouth, lightly suctioned at all times, with the teeth almost closed and the lips closed. This is the ideal mouth posture for breathing, eating, speaking and even facial and dental growth!

This tongue resting posture affects your child's bone development. As the tongue rests against the palate bone, it gently expands the palate bone to get wider. A wider palate means there is more room for teeth. If the tongue is not resting on the palate bone, the bone can grow *up* into the sinus cavity, instead of *out* to make it wider and the child develops a high arched palate. Now it is ever *harder* to rest the tongue on the palate bone, because the palate bone is too high up! Having a high arched narrow palate makes it difficult to clearly produce some speech sounds that require tongue to palate contact, like /l/.

It is important that your child breathes through his nose with his lips closed. Breathing through the nose warms the air, humidifies the air and filters out microorganisms and pollutants from reaching his lungs. It also affects the growth of the facial bones and helps develop the muscles necessary for breathing, chewing, swallowing and speaking.

But then what happens? Toddlers get colds and strep infections. Your child may have allergies and a chronic stuffy nose. This forces him to breathe through his mouth. Now his nose is *not* warming, humidifying and filtering the air, and so the tonsils and adenoids enlarge to take over the job. When a child's mouth is chronically open just to breathe, his jaw is open and his tongue begins to move forward between the teeth and sometimes between the lips. Remember, the tongue is supposed to rest on the roof of the mouth so that the pressure of the tongue muscle expands the palate bone to make it wider. If the tongue is resting forward, the hard palate has the option of growing *up* rather than *out*. In addition to needing orthodontia, your child may lisp, because his tongue is too forward to produce /s/ and /sh/ and /j/ sounds. We see a lot of children in our office who use a forward tongue to produce just about every speech sound. You can observe this in your child – ask him to say daddy, nana and sister – if he you see his tongue coming out beyond his teeth, he has a forward resting tongue posture.

Chronic mouth breathing may change the growth of your child's face. The facial bones can grow longer and there may be dark circles around the eyes. To compound this, children with an open mouth posture are likely to *snore* and develop upper airway resistance syndrome, in which the child has interrupted sleep and all the consequences that brings. So yes, chronic mouth breathing in young children something a parent must be aware of because it is a potential cause of crooked teeth, speech sound disorders, abnormal growth of the palate and the face and chronic susceptibility to infections. This condition is reversible if nasal breathing is restored.

When we see a child with a chronic open mouth and forward tongue, we first refer the child to an allergist to determine if he is congested due to allergies. We want the child to first be able to breathe through his nose. In our office, we are trained in orofacial myology and we work with dentists, orthodontists and ENTs to help a child achieve correct tongue resting posture. We have found through the years that correcting the *posture* makes it easier to correct the *speech,* and this affects the child's entire growth and well-being.

We often get referrals from school speech pathologists for this oral function therapy. In our state, school speech pathologists are required to only address speech and language issues that affect a child's academic performance, and some structural issues don't qualify for school speech therapy. In our private practice, we address issues that affect a child's medical well-being, and we are trained in oral function therapy because it affects a child's general health.

Heather's advice to parents: People are very opinionated, especially family members who don't understand what your child is going through. I got so much flack for following up on what turned out to be structural issues that were affecting Reagan's ability to speak! I was concerned about how all these issues would affect her learning and academics. I think that when you bring your child for an evaluation, there are things that are brought to your attention that you didn't even know were there, and that's a good thing. I shudder to think what would have happened if I had not gotten her the help she needed when she needed it!

I was fortunate to have trusted professionals on my side. But family members can be very opinionated and I think that definitely deters a lot of parents. When you have a gut feeling about your child, you need to get it checked out!

In the next chapters, I'm going to describe two very common structural issues that we see in our office: tongue thrust and tongue tie.

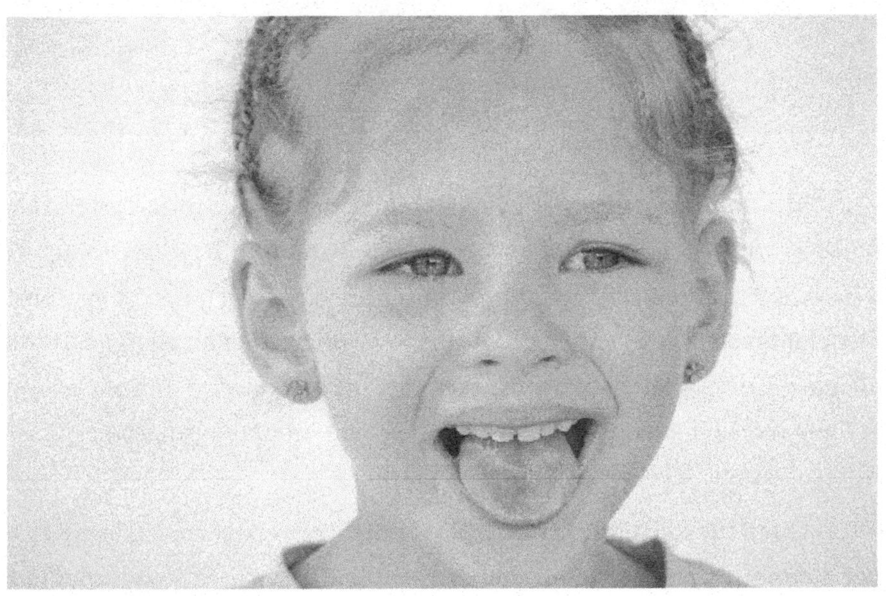

Reason #5 My Child Has a Tongue Thrust

This is Hannah. Hannah is a 4 ½ year old girl who is bright and chatty. There is a gap between her upper and lower front teeth and she usually sticks her tongue in the gap. Her tongue is always forward, and she lisps. Her mother says she will not give up her pacifier.

If your child has a tongue thrust, she is resting her tongue too far forward in her mouth. Two signs of a tongue thrust are an open bite and lisping.

An open bite means that the front teeth don't meet. The teeth have not descended fully because there is something blocking their descent: the tongue! A child with an open bite often rests her tongue through her teeth and her mouth hangs open. As we said, this leads to a cycle of problems.

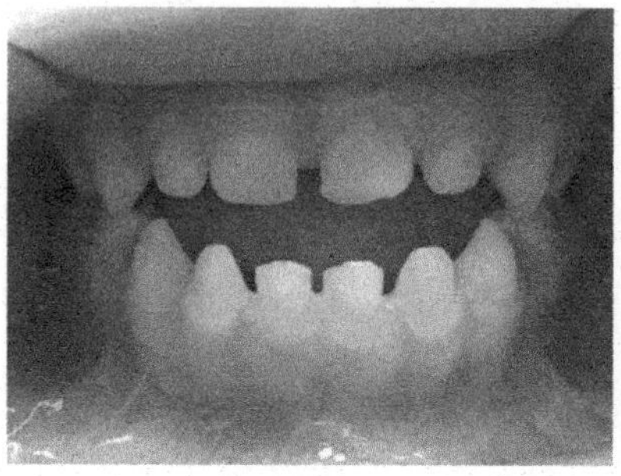 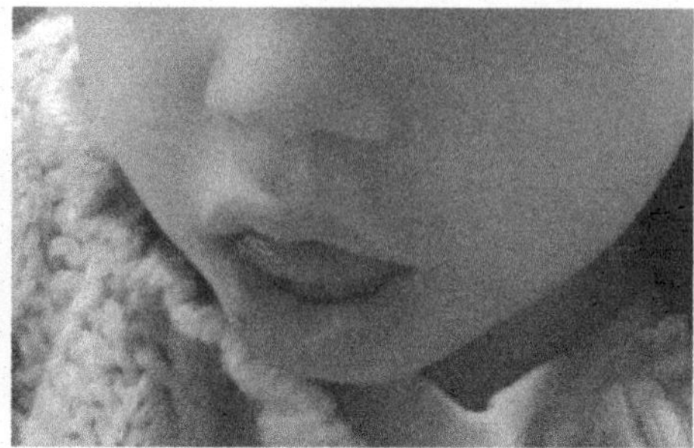

The first thing we assess when a child with a tongue thrust enters our office is *why does he have an open bite, a forward tongue posture and possibly mouth breathing? What started this?* Here are some possible reasons: The child may have allergies and needs to be referred to an allergist. If the allergies are not dealt with first, speech therapy and myofunctional therapy will not work. If allergies are causing the congestion, the congestion must be cured at that level first.

Often the open bite is caused by something very correctable: a pacifier, thumb sucking or a sippy cup. If your child's mouth is always plugged up with a pacifier, the pacifier is *causing* the open bite. The open bite then *causes* the tongue to move forward and the forward tongue will *cause* a tongue thrust, often with an irregular swallow and a lisp.

The best thing you can do as a parent is to gradually wean the child off the pacifier. If your child is 2 years old, start to restrict the pacifier at first to only night time and nap time. During the day, when your child is upset, bring him something else to comfort him. Clean up all the pacifiers in the house and don't make them accessible. Keep the sleepy time pacifier where you have control of it. Some parents gradually snip a bit off the end of the pacifier until it is just not satisfying to the child.

Some parents like to have the "Binky Fairy" come and take the pacifier. When the binky fairy comes, the child goes out for a special treat or gets something in exchange. If this seems like a good idea for your child, you may want to get a one of several books for toddlers giving up a binky, such as Goodbye Binky: The Binky Fairy Story by Sinead Condon.

An open bite can also result from thumb-sucking. The thumb is always in the mouth, preventing the teeth from descending. Sometimes, you can see a thumb-print on the child's palate! Stopping your child from sucking her thumb can be challenging. I recommend a program called Unplugging the Thumb, developed by speech-language pathologists and available at www.orofacialmyology.com. The important thing is to reduce pacifier usage or thumb sucking so that your child's face and teeth develop normally.

Sippy cups can also cause a tongue thrust. I'm sure you love sippy cups. You love them because your toddler can drink in the car or in the house without making any spills.

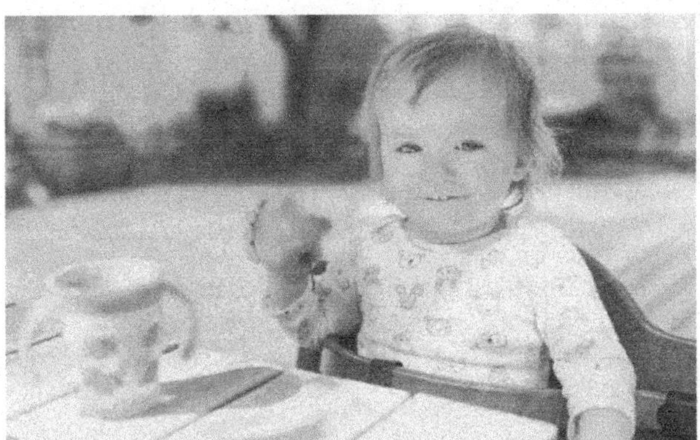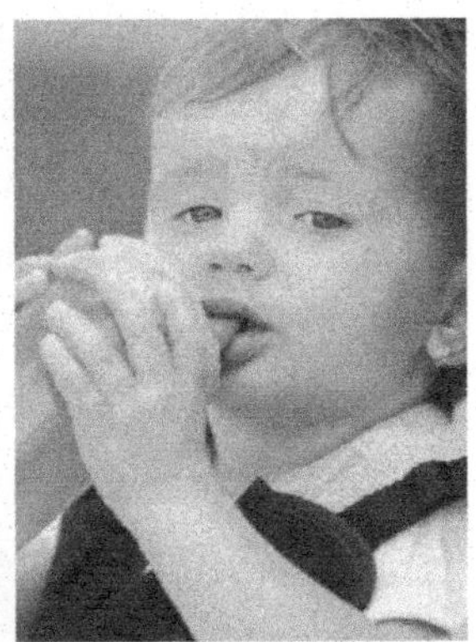

As a parent, it is very important that you choose *the right kind* of sippy cup. The best training cup is one with no valve. Cups with valves do not allow your child to actually *sip* – instead the child is *sucking,* which is an immature way to swallow past twelve months. A cup with a rim or a pop-up straw is better for your child's developing mouth. You still won't have spills, but your child will develop better oral posture. The girl on the left has a sippy cup that contains spills, but does not force her to "suckle" with a forward tongue. The girl on the right has a sippy cup that is more like a bottle. The spout is between her teeth and her tongue comes out under the spout to drink. Over time, these sippy cups cause structural changes in your child's mouth.

It is especially important not to allow children almost total access to sippy cups. Many parents have sippy cups in car and the stroller and children walk around the house drinking all day long. The Journal of the American Dental Association featured an article (2004) warning parents that prolonged bottle and sippy cup use can increase early childhood cavities because the child is using the cup all day.

Speech pathologists who work to correct tongue posture are trained in *myofunctional therapy.* In our office, we help children with tongue thrust develop the correct tongue rest posture for the best growth of the face, the teeth, swallowing and speech. All of these are affected by tongue thrust. Orthodontists refer children to us to achieve correct tongue resting posture, because this greatly affects a child's teeth. A child who keeps her tongue forward and also pushes her tongue forward when swallowing will have an "open bite," which means that her front teeth don't meet. Once the child achieves good tongue posture, there can be a dramatic change in her teeth. Here are some pictures I took recently of a nine- year-old girl who came into our office with a forward resting tongue and a lisp. Five months later, her speech is clear and look at the change in her teeth!

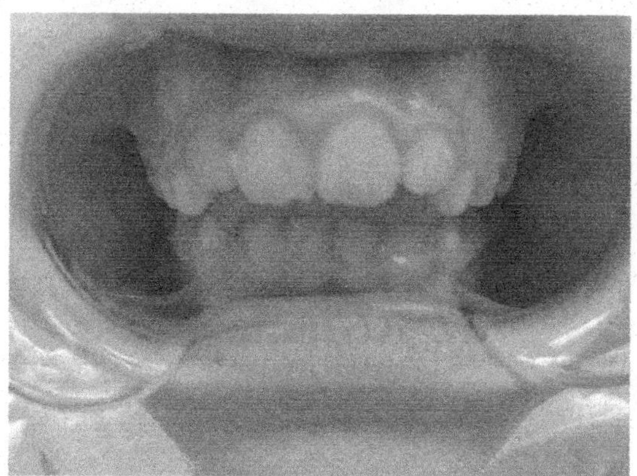
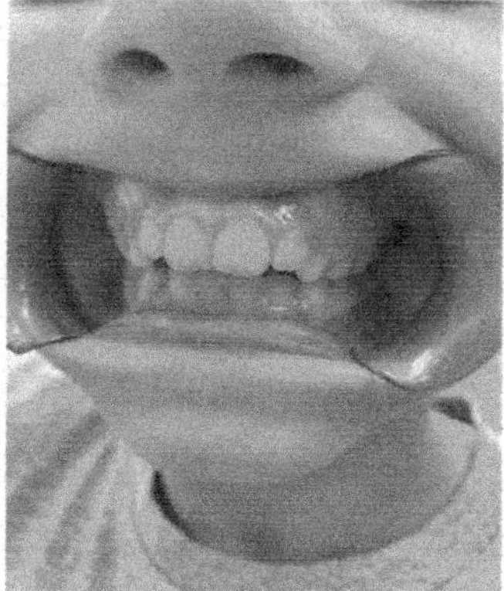

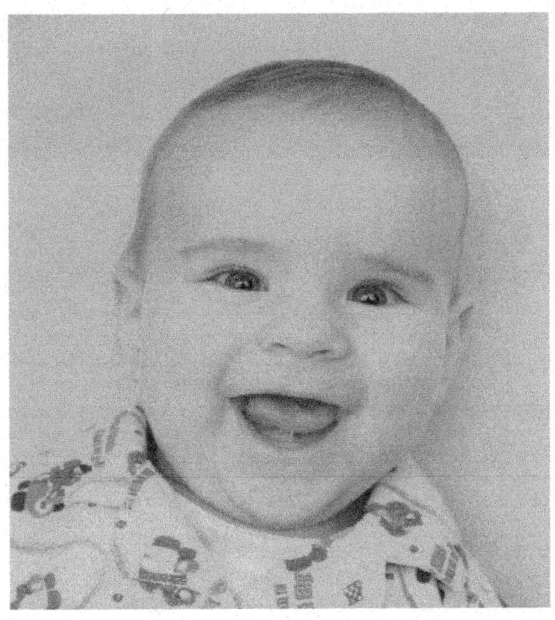

Reason #6 My Child Has a Tongue Tie

This is Cole. Cole was a healthy baby. His mother began breast-feeding him, but he had difficulty latching, so she used a nipple guard. When it became more difficult, she moved to bottle-feeding. As he got older, he began speaking, but no one could understand what he was saying. And his mother complained that he was a very picky eater. "He only eats chicken nuggets and mashed potatoes!" she complained.

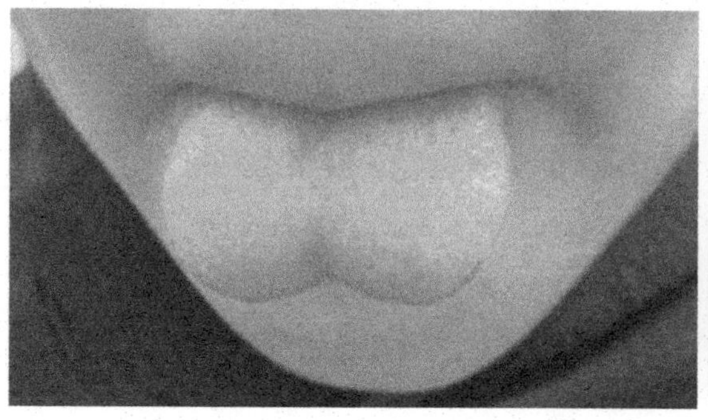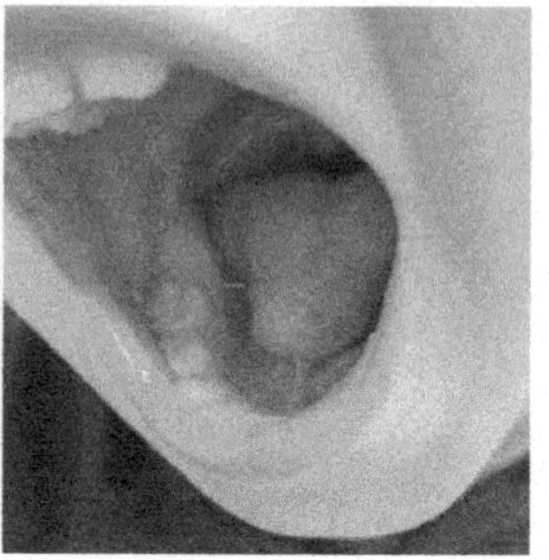

These are pictures I took of Cole's mouth when he came into our office at age four. Do you see how the frenum, the tissue under the tongue that connects the tongue to the floor of the mouth, is too tight? It tethers the front of his tongue to the floor of his mouth. Cole's tongue is heart-shaped because of this and he cannot stick out his tongue or move his tongue around his mouth normally. He also cannot say speech sounds clearly. He could not say words like "alligator" because he could not elevate his tongue to make the /l/ and /t/ sounds, so he said "a-ga-ga".

Cole was diagnosed with a significant tongue tie and was referred to an oral surgeon. After surgery, we helped him learn to move his tongue so that he can speak, eat and swallow properly and clean food off his teeth for dental hygiene. All these functions are affected by a tongue that he cannot move sufficiently.

We often see children who are tongue-tied by a tight or tethered frenum. This is not just a speech issue. A child who is tongue-tied cannot sweep his tongue around his teeth to collect extra food particles left after a meal. A pre-school child came into my office once with 23 fillings in his teeth! It wasn't surprising to find out that he had a tongue tie—he was not able to perform dental hygiene by cleaning his teeth with his tongue.

A tight lingual frenum affects swallowing. This may be discovered early on, when a newborn has difficulty nursing. The child cannot form a seal on the breast because of a restricted tongue. As the child gets older, he needs to elevate his tongue to his palate to swallow correctly, and if this is not physically possible, the child develops an irregular swallow. I have seen children throw their heads back like a bird to swallow, all because the child had a tongue tie and could not propel the food with his tongue! Often, a child with a tongue tie will be a "picky eater" because he cannot handle more advanced textures in his mouth. When you chew food, you use your tongue to move the food from one side to another to thoroughly chew it. A child with a tongue tie cannot do this. A speech pathologist trained in orofacial myology can test for tongue tie and recommend whether the child needs to be referred to an oral surgeon. The diagnosis of a tongue tie is a *functional diagnosis,* meaning that the appearance of the frenum alone does not diagnose a tongue tie. A tongue is tied when the child cannot achieve normal range of motion with the tongue for speech, dental hygiene and swallowing.

Often, correction is a quick laser incision, but sometimes the tongue tie is more complicated and needs oral surgery. A tongue tie can be *anterior,* meaning the tongue is tied in the front, or *posterior,* meaning the tongue tie is further back. A tongue tie must be corrected for normal speech and swallowing. Therapy for tongue tie involves exercises to learn to move the tongue correctly. After the tongue moves correctly, the speech pathologist can focus on producing speech sounds correctly.

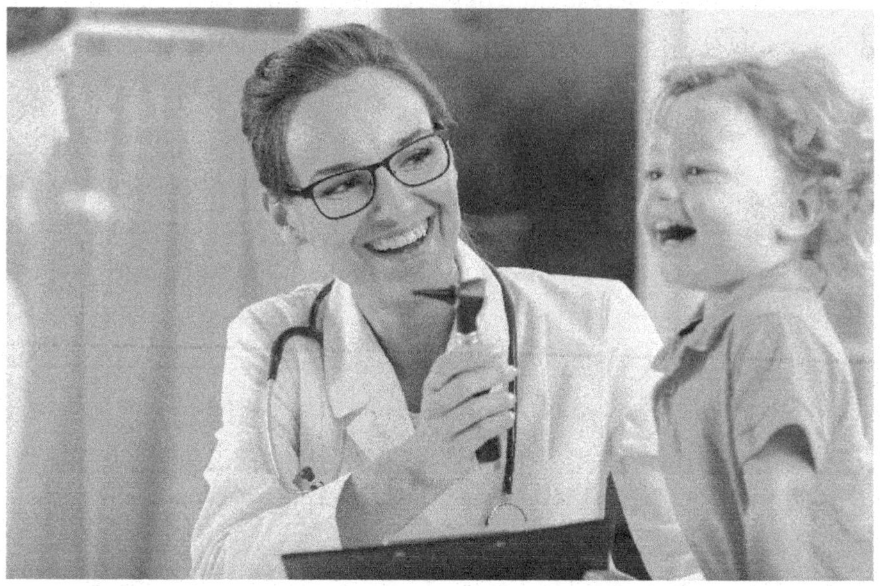

This is Gregory. He is 3 years old. His mother told me this about her son's tongue tie diagnosis:

My son Gregory was approaching the age of 2 and he was not speaking at all. He was doing things that seemed very advanced for his age, but he wasn't speaking. He knew what we were saying and could point to all kinds of pictures, but he could not say any words When he was born, I tried to breast-feed him, but he wouldn't latch. I ended up pumping for many months so he would get my milk. There was talk at that time that he might be tongue-tied, but I didn't know much about tongue tie.

As a baby, Gregory would try to stick out his tongue. My husband and I noticed that we never saw the tip of his tongue. That was the key indicator to us that something was up. I said "Okay, let me bring him to a speech patholo-gist. I came to see you and you said, "I think his tongue is still attached at the very tip" You referred me to the oral surgeon, who agreed with you.

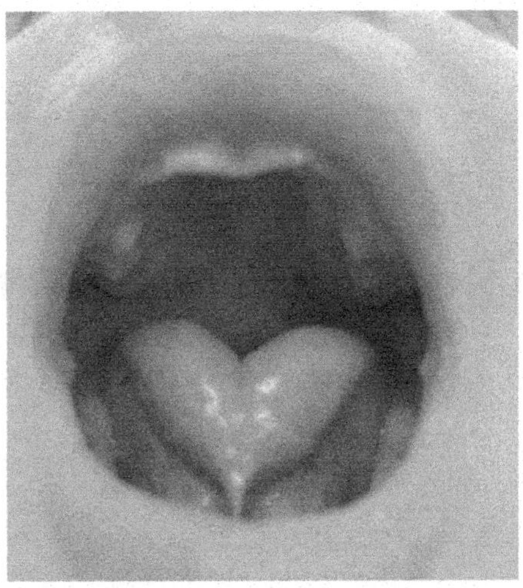

Once I understood why Gregory was not speaking, I really wanted the frenectomy done. I didn't want to hinder him anymore. The only thing that made me nervous for him was going under anesthesia because he was so little. I didn't know if anesthesia would have any effect on his brain. A friend of mine had a son who had tubes in his ears and she reassured me. And, it turned out not to be worrisome after all. Gregory came out of it immediately.

Literally two weeks after he had the frenectomy and started speech therapy, he began to say words! It was wild! People would come up to me on the playground and say, "He's only two and a half? He speaks so well!" They couldn't believe that four months earlier, he couldn't talk!

Now that I'm more educated in tongue tie, I realize it's hereditary. So many of my cousins have children who are tongue-tied. When my second son was born recently, the pediatrician told me he was tongue-tied, but my second son is able to latch and nurse. The tip of Gregory's tongue was attached. My second son has a tight frenum, but the tip is not attached. I'm not going to wait until he is two for a frenectomy. I want to get it done sooner rather than later. With my first son, I didn't know if "tongue tie" was a made-up thing or a fad. Well, it's not made up and it's not a fad. Having a frenectomy and speech therapy changed my son.

11

PHONOLOGICAL PROCESSING

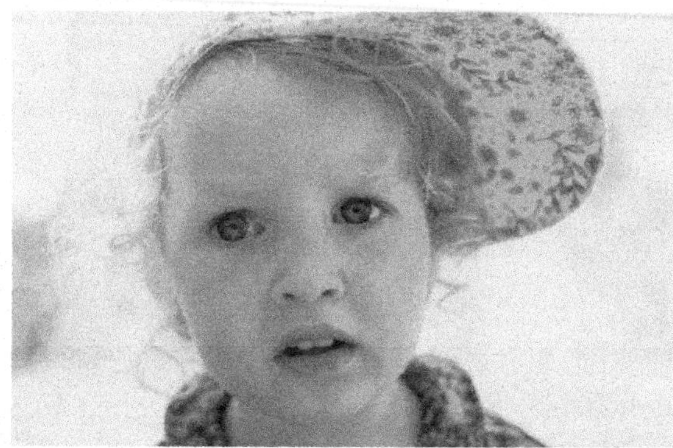

Reason #7: My Child Is Not Perceiving Speech Sounds in Words
A child may *hear* speech sounds but his brain may not *process* the sounds correctly. Often, parents will say, "Oh, he hears well! If a fire truck comes down the street, he runs to the window to see it." Hearing is more complex than simply receiving sounds. Your child may be hearing sounds but his brain may not yet be processing sounds correctly.

It is normal for children to approximate sounds as they learn to speak. For example, a 2-year-old may call a cookie a "tootie." But, at a certain developmental age, a typical child will learn to discern the difference between a "t" sound and a "k" sound and will begin to call it a "cookie."

Children with phonological processing difficulties do not perceive sounds well in words. Sometimes they do not perceive a process, such as making sibilant sounds, which are sounds that force air in a hissing way, such as /s/ and /z/ and /sh/. These children have to be taught how to make sibilant sounds.

Phonological processing disorders are the most common type of speech sound disorders that we diagnose among preschoolers coming to our office. Speech therapy is important for these children prior to beginning kindergarten, because the main goal in kindergarten is to teach children to correlate speech sounds with letter sounds and manipulate them for reading. If your child is not correctly perceiving sounds in words at age 4, learning to read may be very difficult.

Once again, a phonological processing disorder is not a cognitive disorder, but if it is not addressed, the child may have difficulty with reading. I recommend that any child who is four and not speaking all sounds clearly should be evaluated. If there is a phonological processing difficulty and it is addressed in therapy at age four, the child will be much better prepared for kindergarten!

12

MOTOR SPEECH IMPAIRMENT: DYSARTHRIA

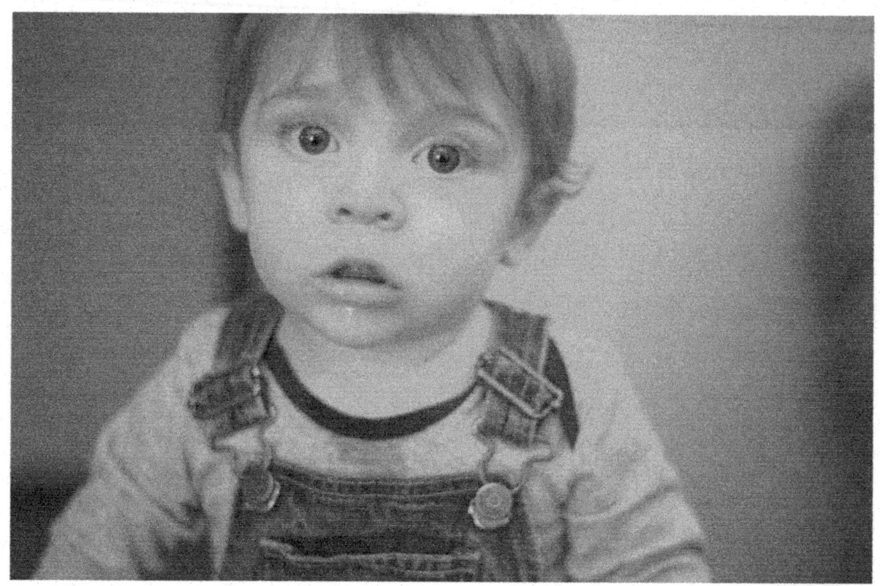

Reason #8: My Child Has Dysarthria

This is Grayson. Grayson is a 3 ½ year old boy who came into the session drooling. His mother said his shirts are always wet. He is not yet able to pucker his lips to "kiss" and his words are difficult to understand. Although Grayson can make almost all consonant sounds once, the longer he speaks, the "mushier" he sounds. Grayson is diagnosed with dysarthria, or muscle weakness.

Dysarthria is caused by impairment in the muscles or the nerves that activate the muscles for speech sounds. A child could have "low tone" in most of his body, or may have "low tone" in just his oral areas. The child's speech will not sound clear, and will be less clear in longer sentences. That is because the muscles are not moving as precisely as necessary. Children with dysarthria often distort speech sounds. Because there is muscle weakness in the oral cavity, a child with dysarthria may be a "sloppy eater" and may also drool.

Dysarthria can be mild, moderate or severe. It often co-exists in children with cerebral palsy, Moebius Syndrome, Down Syndrome and other disabilities. Dysarthria may include difficulty coordinating breathing with speech or moving the jaw, particularly children with cerebral palsy. Some children with dysarthria have involuntary movements called dyskinesias that disrupt their speech. Having dysarthria does not mean that your child has a syndrome, but dysarthria is often one component of a syndrome. Dysarthria is a muscle impairment but is not a cognitive impairment. Therapy for dysarthria usually involves exercises for muscle movements.

13

MOTOR SPEECH IMPAIRMENTS: CHILDHOOD APRAXIA OF SPEECH

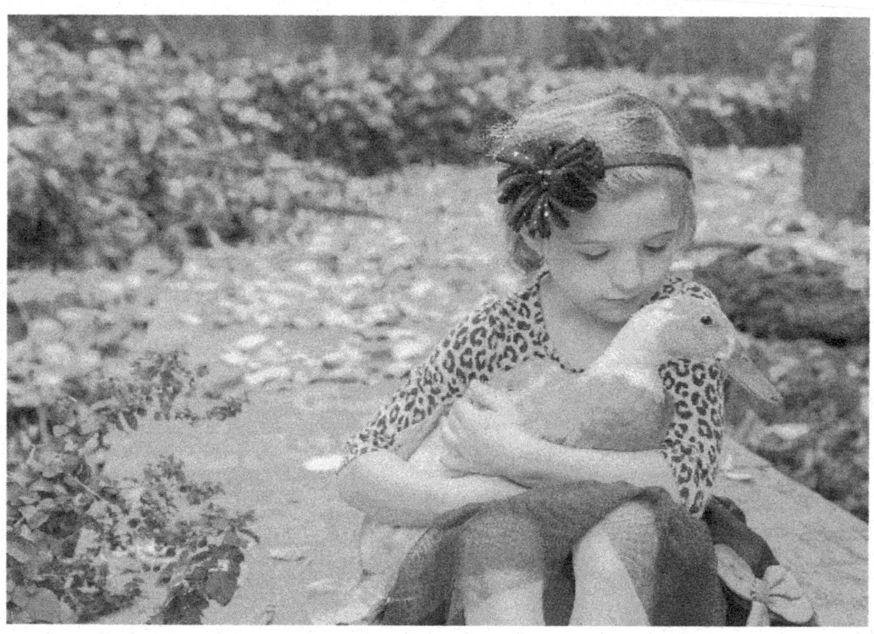

Reason #9: My child struggles with motor planning to produce speech

At age four, Olivia came into our office for an evaluation. It was very difficult to understand what she was saying, because she distorted the vowel sounds in words. Although she could say some simple words, she could not imitate a simple word. I asked her what her favorite animal was. She said "duck." I asked her what her favorite pet was. She said, "duck." I asked her what her favorite farm animal was – it was "duck." What was her favorite ocean animal? "Duck." Olivia was diagnosed from testing as having child-hood apraxia of speech. At the end of the session, I pulled out a roll of farm animal stickers and gave her a duck sticker. She began to cry! It turned out, she really didn't like a duck, but that was the only animal word she could say!

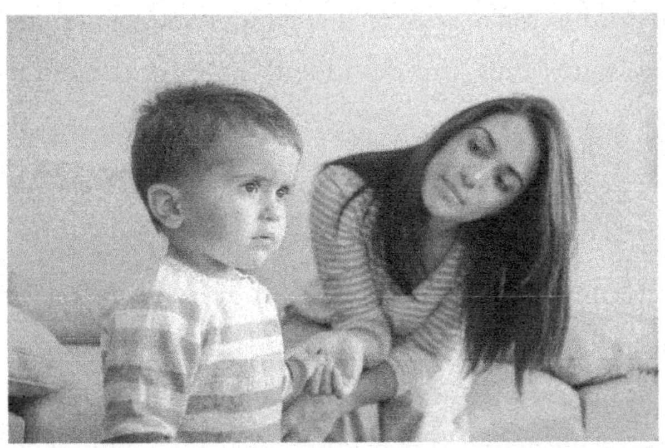

Leo is three. He was a quiet baby, not babbling much and not speaking in jargon. Although he is speaking in sentences now, Leo's speech is choppy, especially on words with more than one syllable. It is more difficult for Leo to say several words than one word. When asked to repeat words, Leo cannot repeat them the same way every time. Leo is having difficulty communicating with others because he has a motor speech impairment. Leo is diagnosed with childhood apraxia of speech.

To produce speech, your child must make rapid motor movements with appropriate intensity in the correct order. This is motor planning. Think of the sequences of motor movements you need to produce a tennis serve – achieving the correct stance, tossing the ball to a spot where you can accurately hit it and swinging the arm with the racquet at the precise moment when you can best hit the ball. Speech is like that, with hundreds of small but accurate jaw, tongue and lip movements coordinated with breath. A child who has difficulty with motor planning may be diagnosed with childhood apraxia of speech.

A child with apraxia knows what he wants to say but cannot achieve the coordination to say it. He may have babbled little as a baby and not said any words by his first birthday. When he did start speaking, the words were short. But, sometimes a child with apraxia will suddenly say a word he has never said before, like "tetradactyl." As his parent, you may be amazed and ask him to say it again, but he cannot. That is because the impairment is in the *volitional* production of speech. It is difficult to *intend* to say a word and then say it, but sometimes, without intent, the word comes out.

A child with apraxia can usually use mouth movements that are not speech-related, such as kissing, chewing and swallowing. The difficulty is motor planning for speech.

A key feature of childhood apraxia of speech is inconsistent production of the same word. For example, the child may sometimes say the word "cookie" as *too-tie* and then say it as *coo-tee* or maybe *oo-ee* but cannot say it the same way repeatedly. This is different from a child who may always call a cookie a *too-tie.*

Another feature of apraxia is that the child may insert *uh* into words inappropriately, such as saying *guh-reen* for "green" or adding *uh* to the end of words, almost giving the child what appears to be an Italian accent! Children with apraxia often distort vowel sounds. They usually do not have difficulty with eating or handling food in the mouth and usually do not drool.

Because children with apraxia have difficulty with the motor patterns for speech, therapy focuses on mastering words with very simple motor patterns, and gradually moving to words with more complex motor patterns. It is usually recommended that a child with childhood apraxia of speech have therapy several times a week with daily practice. Depending on the severity of the apraxia, you may expect therapy to last for a few years. Often, the child will make very significant progress from age three or so until age seven or eight. Therapy will often stop at this time. In my experience, however, there may be periods of speech therapy once or twice again, as speaking demands become more complex as the child gets older. Sometimes, an older child notices that it is difficult to be understood when saying multi-syllabic words or that the intrusive *uh* sound is evident in his speech. I have often worked again with the same child for a year or two, maybe at age ten and again at age fourteen.

A parent who has a child with apraxia can get discouraged and wonder if there will ever come a day when speech therapy is not needed. That day will come and your child will live a normal life if you provide him with the therapy he needs when he needs it.

Parents often call our office, enquiring if we will use the PROMPT program for therapy with their child with apraxia, but this may or may not be the best therapy for your child. There are several approaches that have held up to the research, and as a parent, you should consult with a speech-language pathologist who will suggest the best program for your child.

Years ago, before speech therapy, a child with apraxia of speech would have become an adult with a speech impediment. Today, that does not have to happen.

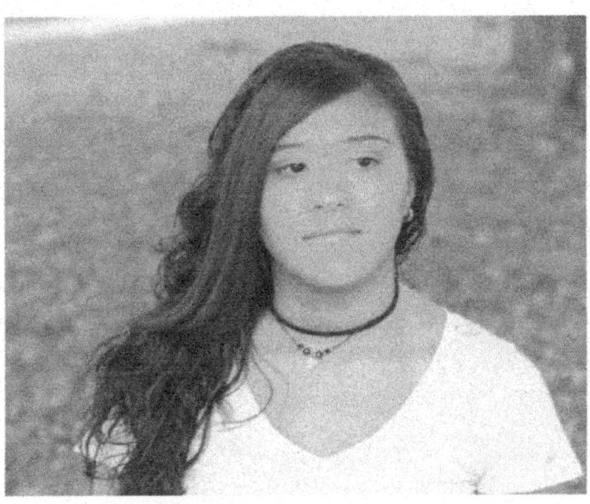

This is Jeanette. Jeanette was 13 years old when I met her. She had normal intelligence, but I could not understand a word she said. She was diagnosed with severe childhood apraxia of speech. Jeanette came from an unstable home life. It appeared that no one was interested in helping this girl practice her speech, which is essential for severe apraxia. She avoided

speaking because she was so ashamed of the way she spoke. It really struck me how important it is to be a diligent parent if your child is diagnosed with childhood apraxia of speech. It makes all the difference in the world! I worked with this teen-ager for almost two years before her family moved again. She was crying when she left and she gave me a bracelet and told me she was so glad someone helped her learn to speak clearly.

14

STUTTERING, CLUTTERING, AND WORD-FINDING

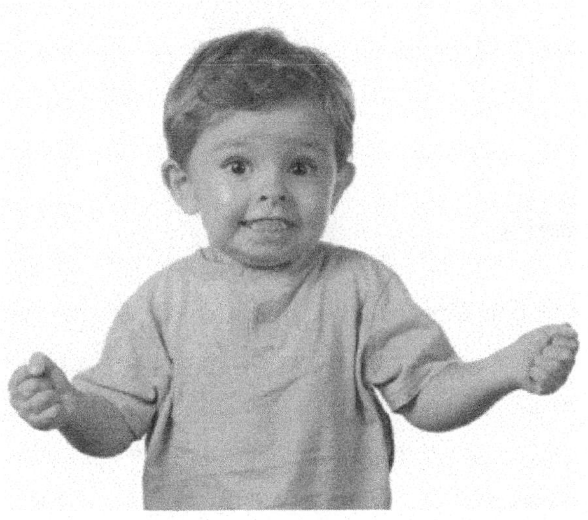

Reason #10: My child stutters

What is dysfluency?

Young children are just learning to talk. Just as toddlers learning to walk often stumble and fall, most young children will not always speak smoothly. Sometimes the child may repeat the first word in a sentence, particularly if the sentence begins with the word "I," as in "*I-I-I-I-I see the puppy!*" Parents notice that this happens most often when the child is very excited or very tired. Some children may have times when they seem dysfluent and other times when they speak more fluently.

A dysfluency is any disruption in the smooth flow of speech. There are three types of dysfluencies that you need know about.

Normal dysfluency is a temporary excitement and is characterized by occasional repetition of whole words or phrases. The child may be excited, but you don't see body tension from the inability to "get the words out."

Some examples would be:

Bobby- Bobby-Bobby jumped in the pool first.

Bobby-Bobby jumped-Bobby jumped in the pool first.

If you notice these types of whole word repetitions, your child may just be going through a normal phase and may become more fluent in a few weeks.

What is stuttering?

Stuttering is the disruption in the smooth flow of speech accompanied by physical tension and struggle. Very importantly, a child who stutters *feels* like he's struggling. He wants to speak and he can't get the words out. A child who stutters usually repeats sounds in words. *"B-b-b-b-b-bobby jumped in the pool first!"* or *"Bobby jumped in the p-p-p-p-pool first."* The child who stutters often has some physical tension and you may notice that he jerks a leg or taps a hand or blinks his eyes when he struggles. He may "block," meaning that he opens his mouth to speak and struggles but there is too much tension for the word to come out. He may be frustrated or embarrassed.

Many children who stutter have developed certain "fear sounds," which are sounds that your child knows to be difficult. If this were, say, the sound of the letter "N," your child will eventually avoid words with the "n" sound, sometimes saying other words in place of the word he wants to speak, or sometimes saying nothing at all, even when he wants to speak. One of my clients told me he wanted to order Nutella ice cream, but he was so afraid of saying "Nutella" in public, he ordered chocolate instead. If this goes on for enough time, your child may become anxious about speaking and will try to avoid speaking situations. This fear of speaking can then affect your child socially and academically.

What is cluttering?

Cluttering is similar to stuttering, but with different characteristics. Cluttering is sometimes called "machine-gun speech" because it comes out in rapid bursts with an irregular rate and includes pauses where pauses are not appropriate. A child who clutters may repeat whole words, often does not finish words and has a lot of filler words, such as *um, well, like.* She sometimes even repeats part of a word, such as *chair-air,* or reduces a multi-syllable word, such as *certly* for *certainly.*

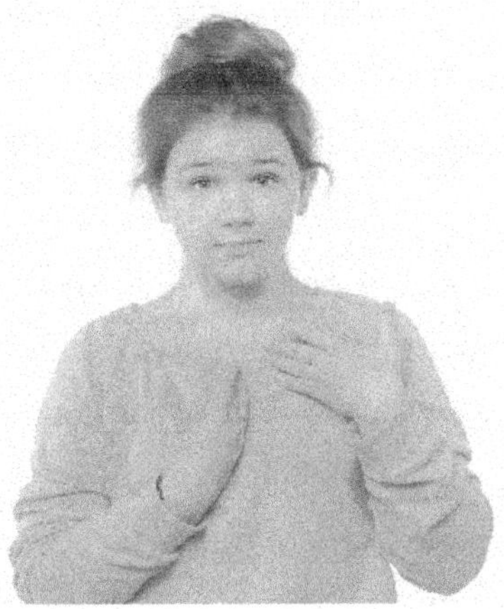

This is Ashley. Ashley is 13 years old and came into our office for a fluency evaluation. This is what she said to me:

We-we-we're learning about, like spe-spe-specific animals like, um, like mine is the …mine's the jaguar. And, and, and we have to write, um, we have to write, like from, like from the animal's perspective but, but we have to write li-li-li-like a diary entry about, about that um, about, about that animal from their, from like, from their perspective and, and each, and each has to include a random fact about the ani-animal like a diary entry.

That is cluttering.

What is word-finding difficulty?

Sometimes, it is not stuttering, but word-finding difficulty that slows down a child's speech A child may know the word he is trying to say, but lacks the ability to *retrieve* the word. Parents may mistake this for stuttering because some of the characteristics are similar.

A child with word-finding difficulty may substitute a word for the target word, saying "cutting" for "knife" but not because he struggles with the /n/ sound, but because he can't retrieve the word "knife" from his brain. He might have a long delay producing a word, but it's not "blocking" because he can't physically get the word out. He might repeat words in conversation, such as "I need to get the, get the, get the…" because he cannot recall the word "knife." He might use fillers such as *um, uh, like* frequently. Word-finding difficulty is not technically a dysfluency, it is language disorder.

A child who is stuttering knows the word he is trying to say, but has physical difficulty getting the word out. A child who has word-finding difficulty does not have physical difficulty getting the word out, he is having language difficulty retrieving the word from his brain. A speech-language pathologist is able to diagnose the difference between stuttering, cluttering and word-finding difficulty.

How common is stuttering?

Research has indicated that up to five percent of people have stuttered at some point in their lives. By adulthood, one percent of the population struggles with fluency, so many children stutter in childhood and achieve fluency later in life. Most children who will eventually be diagnosed with stuttering begin to stutter by age four. Twice as many pre-school boys as girls stutter but by adulthood, there are four times as many males than females who stutter.

What causes stuttering?

Parents often worry that children begin to stutter because of things that happen to them: the family is moving, the parents are separating, a grandparent dies. However, if only stressful situations caused stuttering, then stuttering would be more prevalent in children who grow up in neglectful or abusive homes, which has not been shown to be true.

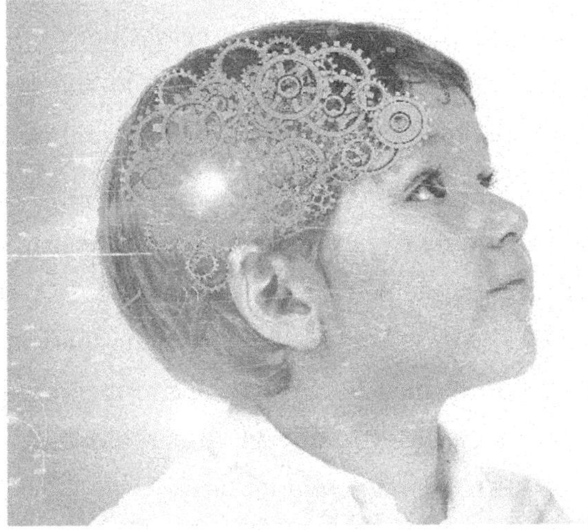

Recent research by Dr. Soo-Eun Chang at the University of Michigan has confirmed that stuttering is a neurodevelopmental disorder. The neural networks that control speech, especially the initiation and timing of speech movements work differently in people who stutter as contrasted with people who don't stutter. Myelin is a substance that speeds up the transmission of nerve impulses in the brain. Some parts of the brain have decreased myelinization in people who stutter. It's not that the brains of people who stutter are different – it's the connections that the neural networks make within the brain that are different.

Genetics plays a role. Researchers have found that 60% of those who stutter also have a family member who stutters. Dr. Dennis Drayna, a researcher with the National Institute of Health, has identified mutations in several genes linked to stuttering.

A team of researchers at Purdue University found that stuttering is a complex disorder on many levels. Family history plays a role but it's not as strong as some other factors. They found that a child who stutters listens to and processes language differently in his brain.

Stuttering isn't caused by stress or anxiety, but stress and anxiety can make it worse. A mild stutter can become severe when the person has to make a telephone call or give a speech. Temperament is not a *cause* of stuttering but can play a role in how the child *responds* to stuttering. Some children may be much more bothered by stuttering than children with different temperaments.

In short, stuttering is a neurodevelopmental disorder with a genetic component in which some parts of the brain have reduced myelinization connecting the neural networks. Part of this is genetic, part is language ability, part is coordination of muscles for speech production and part is auditory processing of language. It is not an anxiety disorder, although anxiety can make it worse. It is complex.

Will my child recover from stuttering as he gets older?

You may have heard people say, "A lot of children stutter. He'll probably grow out of it."

There is a good chance that a young child who stutters will grow out of it. However, the *longer a child stutters, the less likely it is he will grow out of it.* So, the question is, will *your* child grow out of it?

There is much new research on this. Dr. Chang at the University of Michigan investigated whether there are differences in brain imaging in children who continue to stutter versus children who recover. She conducted brain imaging (fMRI) studies of 39 children who stuttered. Over three years, 15 of the children recovered from stuttering and 24 children persisted. The children whose stuttering persisted also demonstrated lower scores than the recovered children in speech motor skills and articulation skills. They were not significantly lower to warrant speech therapy, but lower than the children whose stuttering did not persist. Dr. Chang's research suggests that there are networks that connect attention, speech motor skills, perception, emotion and temperament and children who persist stuttering have differences from children who recover.

At Purdue University, many studies have examined children who persist in or outgrow stuttering. Usler, Smith and Weber in 2017 studied 67 children who were five to seven years old. Several years later, 21 of the children were still stuttering, 15 had recovered and 31 were non-stuttering. Interestingly, the children who persisted in stuttering had more variability in their lip movements at their first visit than the other children. Therefore, according to Dr. Chang's research, these children may have subtle difficulty with muscle coordination for speech.

The researchers concluded that, in general, the motor coordination for speech of children who persist in stuttering is less refined and less mature compared to other children. They hypothesize that children who stuttered but recovered may have overcome a maturity lag in speech motor development.

There is hope. Researchers at the University of Toronto recently published papers on the results of PET scans they took on stutterers. They discovered that the scans showed that speech is a more effortful, less automatic process for stutterers. The stuttering children then participated in an intensive therapy program. One year later, the children were scanned again and researchers found that the stutterers who participated in intensive therapy gained great automaticity in speech from their frequent practice of fluency skills.

Stuttering is complex. A person who stutters knows exactly what he wants to say, but cannot say it at the rate he would like. And sometimes even severe stutterers can speak very fluently. For example, many stutterers can be completely fluent singing or reciting the pledge of allegiance.

We don't fully understand the reasons for this variability. Children may go through periods of dysfluency that can last for days, weeks, or even months. Likewise, they can also go through periods of smooth speech. They may also stutter more or less because of how they think, feel, or react in different situations, or to different people, or to different topics.

Keep this in mind so that you don't think that your child is not working hard enough if he stutters more at times or if you wonder if there's something wrong because his stuttering has gotten worse. Sometimes, stuttering just varies.

Should I make my child aware of his stuttering?

Years ago, people thought that saying the word "stuttering" would increase the likelihood that a child will self-label and continue stuttering. Today, we know that many young children are aware of stuttering. The word stuttering simply describes interruptions in their speech. The more comfortable they become with the term, the less likely they will be to react negatively when other people talk about their speech.

Can stuttering be cured by medication?

There are currently no FDA approved medications to treat stuttering. Interestingly, dopamine blocking medications that have been shown to reduce stuttering. This may support a theory that too much dopamine is a part of what causes stuttering. Dopamine is a neurotransmitter that has an important role in motor control and movement selection, both necessary for speech movement. There were some studies in the 1970's in which stuttering adults were administered a dopamine antagonist, known as Haldol.

Haldol works by blocking dopamine receptors in the brain. The studies concluded that Haldol was more effective than placebo in promoting fluency. However, many participants in the study dropped out because the negative side effects of Haldol were too extreme and sometimes resembled Parkinson's disease.

Can speech therapy cure stuttering?

No. A speech pathologist can help your child manage stuttering, but cannot *cure* stuttering.

Early treatment for stuttering helps your child speak as smoothly as possible. There are several approaches to stuttering therapy, and your speech pathologist will choose the one that appears to best fit your child. Most treatment methods center around reducing *tension* during speech and *timing* breathing with speech.

Importantly, speech therapy gives children techniques to use when they find themselves stuck when they're trying to speak. Some of the techniques, such as using an easy onset breath when starting to speak, will allow a child to manage socially. Often in speech therapy we practice situations which can be challenging for people who stutter, such as making a phone call. We have done things like calling local businesses to ask what time they are open today. After a session of practice, the fear of making a phone call has lessened.

After age 7, it becomes unlikely that stuttering will go away completely. Still treatment can be very effective at helping a child manage stuttering, such as developing the skills necessary to handle difficult situations like teasing or bullying, and to participate in school activities. For older children, speech therapy helps reduce the severity and impact of stuttering. What works for one child may not work for another child for various reasons. Therapy needs to be tailored to the child who walks in the door, not one program slapped on children in a study.

My child may be stuttering if he:

* Repeats initial sounds in words

* Shows tension when trying to speak

* Has secondary symptoms when speaking, such as blinking, twitching, tapping a leg

* Opens his mouth to speak, but no words come out

* Tells you that speaking can be difficult

STUTTERING *A fluency disorder*	CLUTTERING *A fluency disorder*	WORD-FINDING *A language disorder, not a fluency disorder*
Speaking includes physical tension or struggle	Rapid bursts of speech	Pauses in speech because can't pull up the word
Repeats sounds within words, usually the first sound	Repeats parts of words or whole words	A long delay before producing a word, but without physical tension
Words appear physically blocked from coming out	Pauses in the wrong places	Frequently adds filler words
Avoids words with "fear sounds"	May reduce or not finish multiple-syllable words	
Adds secondary movements or filler words to help get the word out		

For Parents:

How Do You Look at Your Child?

Be aware of how you look at your child while he speaks. The look on your face can either add to his fear of speaking, or it could encourage him to speak. It might be helpful to look in the mirror and pretend your child is stuttering. What message does your face tell him? Remember that stuttering is not his fault, nor is it your fault—it's just how he speaks.

Yes-or-No Questions

Do not ask your child a question when you're rushed for an answer. If you need an answer quickly, ask him a yes-or-no question so he can answer by nodding or shaking his head. This eliminates stress when people are rushed.

Allow Time to Speak

Allow your child the time to speak during family conversations. If you have some family members who speak fast or who may not listen well, talk together as a family on how you can improve listening skills and provide positive interactions so that the child who stutters has time to talk and feels like a valued part of family conversations.

Provide Positive Speech Experiences

Allow your child the opportunity to read out loud to a pet, if you have one. Some libraries have trained, calm therapy dogs who will sit next to a child and just listen. Reading out loud to another human can feel scary, but a child will often stutter far less when reading aloud to an animal. This kind of practice will build confidence so the child can eventually read aloud before people. Find and repeat any positive speech experience.

Teach Self-Compassion

A child who stutters can often be very hard on himself and "play" his speech over and over in his mind. He may get angry or frustrated but it is because he is angry at himself or his situation - not you. Teach him self-compassion. Show him how to observe his stutter without judging his worth or status in life. Instead of thinking "Oh, no! This is so embarrassing, what will people think?" he could think "Interesting…I'm stuttering right now. It's okay. This doesn't make me less of a person. It's just something unique about me." You can help you child learn how to feel good about who he is with stuttering as part of his life.

Prevent Isolation

Find communities for your child to meet other kids who stutter. Stuttering is often very isolating for a child. Any situation where he feels accepted and less alone will be helpful. He can find this kind of acceptance when he meets someone else who stutters, whether it is in person, online, or through a book.

Many children's books help frame stuttering as something to manage—not something to be ashamed of. These are some great examples:

"I Talk Like a River" by Jordan Scott

"When Oliver Speaks" by Kimberly Garvin

"Unstuck" by Stephen Groner

Katie, now a book editor and a mom, tells what it was like growing up stuttering:

I started stuttering in elementary school and it felt like something was wrong with me. I was embarrassed and ashamed. I went to speech therapy because I thought my speech disappointed my parents. I wish I could have gone to speech therapy without having to worry about my parents. The speech therapists at my schools were helpful, and if nothing else, they provided a safe spot for me in what felt like a war zone.

I highly recommend any kind of speech therapy for a person who stutters. School was tough. I quickly learned how to edit everything I would say before I ever said it. I avoided certain letters or words, I even avoided specific situations. I avoided anything that would make my stuttering worse. I just wanted to speak like everyone else. Many assumed I was not smart or could not read, when in fact, I was an avid reader. I just didn't read out loud.

I left my classroom to attend speech therapy, and it was always embarrassing to come up with various stories about where I went when friends would ask. Eventually, my sixth-grade teacher explained to our class that I was attending speech therapy and to stop asking me. She also let them know that I would be excused from reading out loud unless I wanted to. These two things made my school life suddenly so much easier. School finally became a place I liked, not a place where I felt constant fear and panic. I had one junior high teacher who let me give an oral presentation in front of only her after school, instead of in front of the whole class. By the end of the year, I was able to give my presentations in front of the class.

I met with a speech therapist at that junior high, but it was during P.E., so most of the time, no one knew that I was missing. As I got into high school and continued finding flexible teachers, I gained more confidence with my speech. I think much of my stuttering stemmed from the panic of worrying that I would stutter. When people showed me flexibility, understanding, and a lack of judgment, I was able to have positive speech experiences. Once I had more positive speech experiences than negative ones, I was able to stutter a lot less frequently.

I eventually overcame the fear of speaking and reading out loud, but I still stutter to this day. I am now 47 years old. I still avoid certain word combinations, certain letters, etc. I still self-edit everything I will say seconds before I say it to ensure that I can say it smoothly. I'm still unable to express opinions around people who talk fast because I know I won't be able to keep up. I haven't tried to learn another language, even though I would really like to do that.

For most of my life, I have judged my stutter harshly and let it determine what I was capable of, what groups of people I talk to, and what careers and talents I pursued. I wish I would have learned earlier in life how to observe my stutter like I would observe my hair color, or the way I walk, or how fast I can run, or my accent. Stuttering is just how I speak.

PART III

What Can I Do to Help My Child?

15

WHERE CAN I FIND HELP?

If your child is struggling with speech or language, it is time to get help.

Fortunately, you have many options. Some of the options may be free, some may be covered by medical insurance and some may involve co-pays.

A child under the age of three is eligible to be evaluated by Early Intervention. Early Intervention is a federally funded program designed to identify and help babies with developmental delays. You can call your local Early Intervention number and, after you give written permission, they will send a team of developmental specialists to your home. The team will observe your child, measure your child's development in specific areas, such as language comprehension, speaking and walking, and they will write a report outlining how your child is functioning in each area. If your child tests a least two standard deviations below the mean in one area of development (such as speaking) or 1.5 standard deviations below the mean in two or more areas (such as speaking and walking or speaking and cognitive development) your child qualifies for services from Early Intervention. Or, if your child is not showing signs of a developmental delay, but has a diagnosed medical condition with a high probability of delays, your child will qualify for Early Intervention Services. For example, if your child is diagnosed with Down Syndrome, there is a high probability of a developmental delay, so your child may qualify for Early Intervention services.

Early Intervention will develop an Individualized Family Service Plan that outlines which services they will provide for your child. They deliver services in the child's natural environment, which means in your home or in daycare. The cost of services is calculated on a sliding scale, based on your income and the number of people in your family.

The purpose of Early Intervention is to ensure that children receive the services they need for appropriate development, whether or not their parents can afford the services. However, the services are not free for everyone. If you have a higher income, Early Intervention services can be more costly than going to private speech therapy using medical insurance.

A private speech-language pathologist can also provide an evaluation and therapy services for your child. Many private services accept medical insurance.

In most cases, Early Intervention delivers services in your home and a private speech language pathologist delivers services in an office.

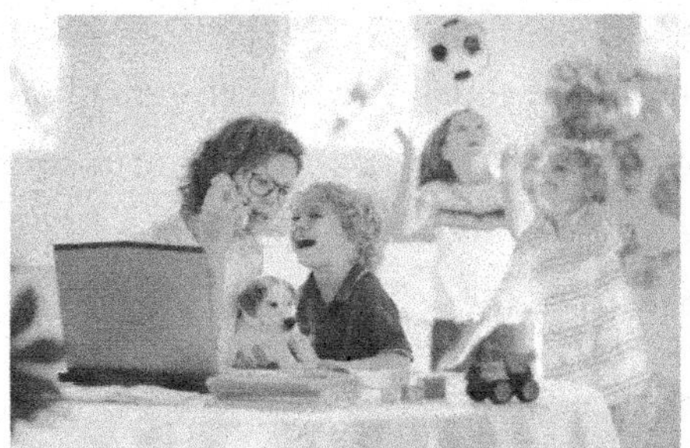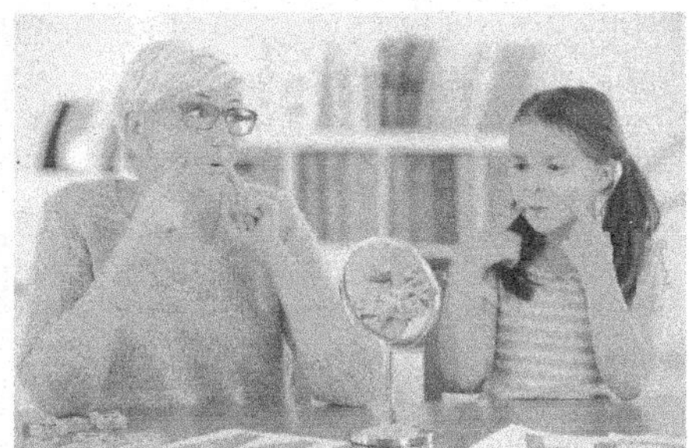

I have provided services in both environments. I believe services in the office are more effective.

In my experience, the home environment can be very distracting. The baby is sitting in the high chair in the kitchen for therapy. The dog is running around barking and the phone is ringing. Grandpa has the television volume turned up in the living room and he's smoking a cigarette. The therapist must compete with all these distractions for the child's attention.

A speech therapy office is a quiet environment where the therapist can more easily get and maintain the child's attention. In our office, we put away all the toys except for one to focus the child's attention. There are no siblings vying for the child's attention and we can get the child to focus on sounds and words because there are no distractions.

Most children really love coming to therapy in our office. They thrive on the one-on-one attention and the upbeat, fun atmosphere. They enjoy the prestige of "going to speech class."

If your child is over the age of three, he does not qualify for Early Intervention any more. Your options are your local school district and private speech therapy. In some communities, there is a college with a speech pathology program and the college may offer low-cost therapy using students to work with your child.

Your three-year-old may be eligible for special education services at the local public school. When you contact your local school district, you will be referred to the Child Study Team. On this team are several professionals, including a speech-language pathologist. The team will get your written permission to do an evaluation of your child's development in several areas. If your child demonstrates significant delay in one or more areas, your child may qualify for the pre-school disabled program. The team, along with you, will put together an Individualize Education Plan, or IEP.

The IEP describes your child's goals and objectives, and details of services needed by your child. The services must be appropriate for your child and must provide a meaningful educational benefit. The cost of the services is covered by the school district and are offered in the Least Restrictive Environment. The least restrictive environment means that if your child can reasonably participate in a classroom with other children, your child will be placed in that classroom rather than, perhaps, a special school for children with autism. However, if your child has severe behavioral issues, then the least restrictive environment for your child might be a school that features intensive intervention for behavioral issues.

It is important for you to know that YOU are part of your child's Child Study Team. Nothing will be done without your permission, and you are able to make suggestions for your child. The Child Study Team will consider your suggestions, and your child may or may not be eligible for what you request. For example, if your child has severe behavioral issues due to a diagnosis of autism, you may request that your child go to an intensive program for preschoolers with autism, rather than attend the pre-school handicapped class. If you request it, it must be considered by the team, but it may not be approved by the team.

Your state may have a pre-school program in a high quality, state-approved private special education school. If the Child Study Team recommends a specialized school for your child, tuition and transportation are paid for by the school district.

If your child has a significant disability, she may make more progress in a school with expertise in educating children with this disability. For example, I once evaluated a four-year-old girl with cerebral palsy who was non-verbal. Her school district suggested the school's pre-school disabled class, but her parents requested a special school for children with severe speech disabilities. The school district agreed to a one-year placement. This little girl went to the special school 5 days a week and received intensive speech therapy by a speech-language pathologist who worked exclusively with children with cerebral palsy. I re-evaluated the girl for the school district a year later. Her progress was truly amazing!

Once your child is kindergarten-age, if your child needs services and you want to go through the public school system, you must request an evaluation be done. If your child only has speech issues, such as stuttering or articulation difficulties, the school's speech-language pathologist will call you to arrange for a speech evaluation. If your child is found eligible, he may qualify for an *Individual Speech-Only IEP*. If your child needs services in more than one area, the Child Study Team will evaluate your child and he will get an Individualized Education Plan, or *IEP*.

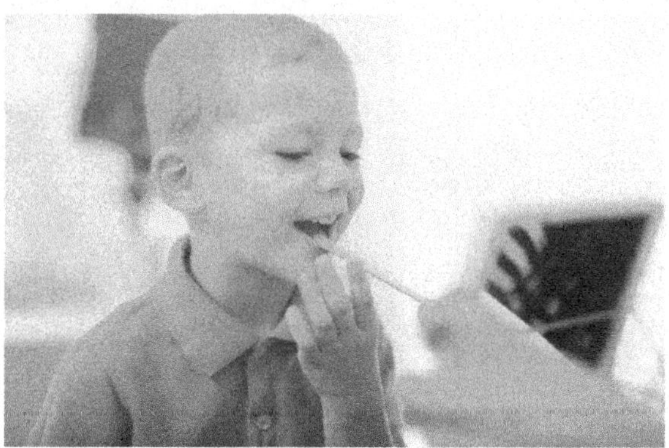

Why should I consider private speech therapy for my child?

There are several reasons why parents prefer private speech therapy. The first reason is that the therapist's entire attention is on your child. Some school districts prefer the "push-in" model where the speech pathologist is asked to sit in the classroom and help the child function with his goals while the lesson is being taught. I have done this in the past. I didn't feel that I was able to work on the child's individual goal as intensively as if I had the child in a quiet room focused on his goal. For example, a child with a lisp needs a quiet environment to hear the sibilance of /s/. That's hard to do in a noisy classroom.

Private speech therapy can be more affordable to parents of a certain income level than Early Intervention. Early Intervention charges a percentage of your income for services. If your medical insurance covers speech therapy, you will pay your normal co-pay for services, regardless of your income. This could be less than Early Intervention!

Medical Goals differ from Educational Goals

You have to understand that medical insurance covers services for *medical goals*. The school district covers services for *educational goals*. There can be a difference. For example, we frequently see children with a tongue thrust and a lisp. These children will often not qualify for speech therapy in the school because having a tongue thrust and a lisp does not affect their *academic performance.* Yet, from a medical perspective, having a forward tongue posture at rest and for swallowing affects the growth of the palate bone, the efficiency of the swallow, the development of the teeth and the production of sibilant sounds. A private speech pathologist may be more trained in correcting the entire problem and she corrects these issues on a daily basis. The school speech pathologist may not be permitted to be trained by the school system in tongue thrust because the school district says this does not have an academic impact.

A child with cognitive delays and language delays may benefit from a school program because these delays affect his *educational goals.* Many school speech pathologists have developed expertise in helping children achieve their educational goals with language therapy.

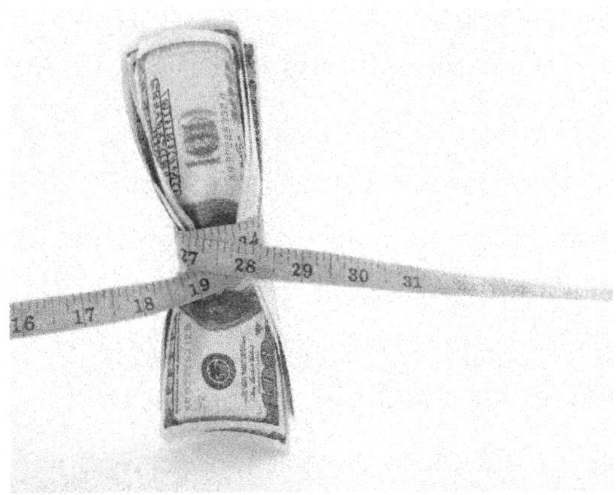

Will my medical insurance cover the cost of private speech therapy?

Maybe. It depends upon what your medical plan covers and your child's diagnosis. Here is how medical insurance works with regard to speech therapy:

If you have a plan with a major medical carrier, such as Blue Cross Blue Shield, Aetna, Cigna or United, your employer has chosen a particular "package" with that insurer. They offer various levels of coverage and your employer may have chosen Package A, B or C. Some packages will not cover speech therapy services, some will cover services for only certain diagnoses and some may cover any diagnosis. A few medical carriers offer unlimited speech therapy, but many medical carriers offer 30 visits or 60 visits a year.

Along with the coverage are the conditions that the insurer will cover. In our experience, the speech and language evaluation is almost always covered by medical insurance. The evaluation concludes with the speech language pathologist's diagnosis. The diagnosis comes with a medical code that lets the insurance company know why services are requested. For example, a child who had continuous ear infections in infancy and missed the critical period for perceiving sounds in words due to hearing loss at that time would receive the code F80.4 speech/language delay due to hearing loss.

Just as many school districts will not provide services for a child without an "educational need," many insurers will not cover services for what they consider "educational needs." Insurance companies often exclude diagnoses due to "developmental delay." If your child needs speech therapy due to a medical reason, it is more likely to be covered.

Sometimes a child can receive school services and private speech therapy if his needs are both medical and educational. Many parents like to supplement school services with private one-on-one services for their child.

If your child's diagnosis is covered under medical insurance, you must still observe the rules of your particular medical plan. You may have a deductible, which is the amount of money you must pay before your medical insurance kicks in. Most deductibles begin every year on January 1st. Many families choose a high deductible plan because the higher the deductible, the lower the monthly charges for insurance. Usually, you must pay for *all medical services* until you reach the amount of your deductible.

A deductible is usually *per person* and *per family.* If your deductible is $500 per person and $2,500 per family, Johnny's speech therapy will not be paid for by medical insurance until Johnny's medical expenses exceed five hundred dollars *or* the family's expenses exceed two thousand five hundred dollars. If Dad had his appendix out on January second and it cost three thousand dollars, the family pays the $2,500 and the family's deductible is met. Insurance kicks in for the rest of the year.

If the family has not yet paid $2,500, they would have to pay $500 in medical expenses for Johnny before speech therapy is covered. Suppose Johnny went to the pediatrician for $100 and the emergency room for stitches. He may have already exceeded $500 for the year and speech therapy would be covered from the first session. If you have not paid $500 towards Johnny's medical expenses this year and he is approved for sixty speech therapy session, you must pay for the first several sessions until you reach $500 and then insurance will pay for the remaining sessions.

In addition to deductibles, most insurance plans have a co-pay. This is the amount you must pay per session while the insurance company pays the rest. If you have a $20 co-pay, you must pay this for each therapy session.

Some families are lucky enough to have a Health Savings Account or Flexible Spending Account; This is a credit towards medical costs not covered by the major medical carrier. You can often use your credits in an HSA or FHA to covers the cost of speech therapy.

Parents have come to us and asked us to "change the diagnosis codes to qualify a child for speech therapy. We are not ethically able to do this. A speech language pathologist is a state-licensed health care provider and is ethically bound to correctly diagnose a speech disorder based on the assessment results. Parents have also asked us to "waive the co-pay," but we are not ethically permitted to do this.

Parents also ask us why we accept some insurance plans and not others. The reason is the reimbursement. The insurance companies set a rate that they will reimburse us for each session. If their rate is too low, we cannot pay our therapists plus overhead if we worked for that rate, so we cannot accept patients with that insurance. However, there are instances in which we can give a receipt of payment to the parent. Then the parent can submit the receipts to the insurer for out-of-network benefits and receive something back from the insurance company.

Sometimes the parents of a child with a significant speech disorder find that their plan does not cover their child's diagnosis. We recommend that you speak with your HR Manager. There are instances in which the HR manager can find a way to cover the diagnosis.

The important thing to remember is that there *is* a way to get your child help. Call your medical insurance company and find out what they cover for speech therapy. Call Early Intervention if your child is younger than three, or your school district if your child is at least three and find out if your child qualifies for services. You can even call the nearest university that has a speech pathology program and find out if their clinic is available for your child. Your child is counting on you!

How am I doing getting help?

Check list for Parents:

* For a child under age three, I have contacted a private speech language pathologist or Early Intervention for an evaluation

* If my child qualifies for services, I have decided whether to have services provided in the home with Early Intervention or with a private speech therapy clinic.

* If my child is over three, I have contacted a private speech language pathologist or my local school district to find therapy services for my child.

* My child has received a diagnosis and I understand why my child is struggling and what the goals are to help my child

* I have called my medical insurance carrier to determine if speech therapy is a covered service. I understand what my deductible and co-pay are for my medical insurance and I have inquired how many sessions per year are covered.

FAQ'S

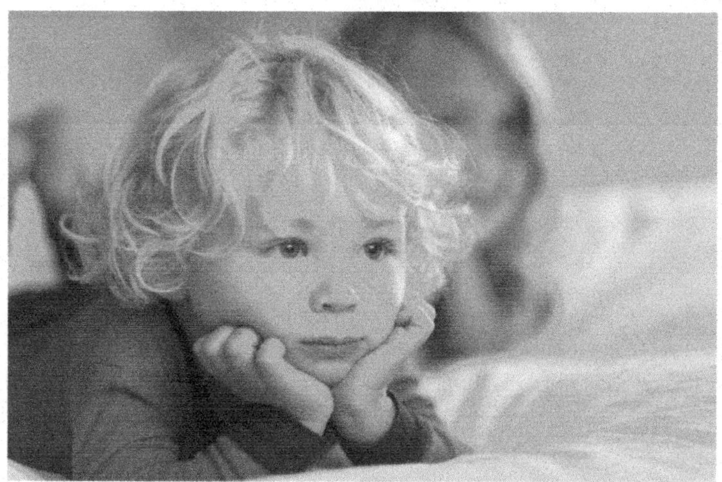

Does Screen Time Affect Speech/Language Development?

I am not opposed to screen time. I raised five children and I know that parents sometimes need a break. And, watching television or a video gives the child's mind access to other worlds and fuels the imagination.

What is important is that screen time be *age-appropriate, focused* and *limited* to certain times of the day. The average American pre-school child spends 32 hours a week watching television. If the child has a television in his bedroom, he averages an extra 90 minutes of more television per day. Two-thirds of American households have the television on during dinnertime. The American Academy of Pediatrics recommends that no children under the age of two should have screens, iPad or television watching. Children over two should have no more than two hours per day of television.

Young children are learning how to process sounds into foreground and background sounds. They can't filter sounds yet the way an adult can filter. A television constantly on in the background is very distracting to a young child and truly hinders the child from paying attention to foreground noise, such as your voice when you call your child.

When I was raising young children, they were permitted to watch children's television shows while I made breakfast. Some of the shows were enchanting, such as Dumbo's Flying Circus, about a group of animals that ran a circus. There was a cat named Lily in the show who walked a tight rope. The kids used to take an umbrella and walk the landscape ties around our house, pretending to be Lily.

In the afternoon, we went out for fresh air, often to the park. When we returned home, they were permitted to watch a video while I prepared dinner. I felt that the videos provided an enriching glimpse of a fantasy land for the children – a land of dinosaurs, princesses, castles, or animals being rescued. Yes, I know parents are told to watch television *with* the child, but my children were watching television so that I could make dinner! It was also down-time for the children after active-time. There was a time for reading books and a time for talking at the dinner table and a time for running in the park with other children. Their television time was my time to get a break! Today they are all educated and employed, so I don't think it did them any harm.

I don't believe it's appropriate to have television or hand-held video games distracting the family at the dinner table. It's during interaction with the family that children learn conversation skills. As a speech pathologist, I always note the sub-skills that a child has acquired for conversation: introducing a topic, maintaining a topic, taking conversational turns and closing a topic. Your child will learn these skills from participating in conversation with older children and adults.

A positive learning experience to be garnered from children's shows and movies is that it subtly teaches narrative structure, which is necessary for expressive language. Narratives have an underlying structure or formula that we understand when we tell stories. For example, if I told you this story: "I went to the store and bought bread. I toasted the bread, then I washed my plate," I am telling you a sequence of events, but it is missing a narrative structure; it's boring! A narrative structure includes an actor with a motive and a challenge, or it's not a story. Instead, if I said, "It was Bobby's fourth birthday and I promised I would make his favorite dinner. He wanted tuna fish on toast. I had cans of tuna, but when I went to the store, there was no bread! They said the bread truck broke down and they wouldn't have bread until tomorrow. What could I do? He would be so disappointed!" Well, that's more of a story! There is a reason for the actions. Children's shows introduce children to narrative structure so that children recognize that actions are goal-oriented. That is why I believe high-quality age-appropriate shows can be very beneficial for pre-school children.

As most parents have learned, once you let a child start video game, it can become an obsession. Please limit time spent on video games! If a child is playing too many video games, what is he not doing? He's missing developmental play. Too much television and video game playing, combined with little developmental play may hinder your child's learning overall. We very often see boys, especially, come into our office with limited expressive language abilities. I wonder how much of it is related to excessive video-game playing, since I have noticed that these boys often spend hours upon hours every week engaged in solitary video game playing!

My daughter, who is a speech pathologist, worked in a school in an economically disadvantaged neighborhood. Most of the children she worked with had delayed language. When she did language evaluations on the children in September, most of the children showed no growth since

June. She would ask the children what they did over the summer. Most of them said "Watch tv" or "played video games." She asked, "Did you go to the beach? Did you have a picnic? Did you go to the zoo?" and the answer was always no, they just watched tv and played video games. Obviously, the television and video games were not enriching enough to show any growth in twelve weeks of summer vacation!

Does Attending Daycare Benefit or Harm Speech Development?

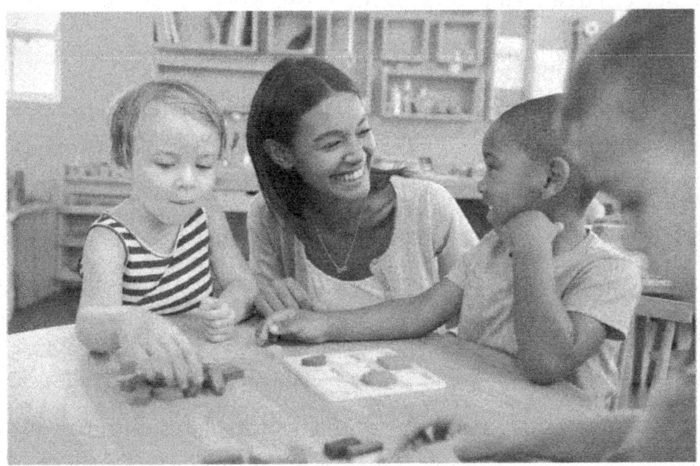

So many parents tell me that they are worried that their child's speech is delayed because he went to daycare….or didn't go to daycare.

I visit many daycares and pre-schools in my area. Our team screens children for speech/language difficulties in many of the local pre-schools. A few are atrocious. Many are truly excellent.

I think it is important that the child receive high-quality care, whether at home or at daycare. His speech and language learning can thrive in either setting. If you are in a position to provide high-quality care at home, with opportunities for the child to regularly go outside and run around, and opportunities to be spoken to individually and with opportunities to play with other children, your child with thrive. One of my own children never went to pre-school because there was too much going on at home at the time. She is a speech-language pathologist today, so it obviously didn't hinder her speech development!

If you are choosing a pre-school or daycare, do spend the time looking for a quality program. You wouldn't think people who found children irritating would run a daycare center, but I recall waiting in the hall to meet with a director. I heard her, in a mean tone of voice, ream out a three-year-old for something relatively minor. When she realized, I was quietly waiting to meet with her, she appeared sheepish, but nonetheless, this is not a high-quality environment for a child.

I have also been asked to screen children in some very filthy rooms, and the child care workers did not seem to realize that they should clean the tables before snack time. I asked for cleanser and paper towels to clean the grimy table before working on it, and the daycare workers told me they didn't have paper towels. The children in this setting did not appear joyful.

But many daycares are a source of joy to young children. A kind-hearted, well-educated director with trained child care workers cast a net of happiness over a school and you can see that the children are growing and glowing. Your child could thrive in this environment, too.

The take-away is that the *quality* of care a child receives matters. A child who is encouraged to develop in a loving, high-quality environment will thrive.

My child receives speech therapy. What is the best way to practice at home?

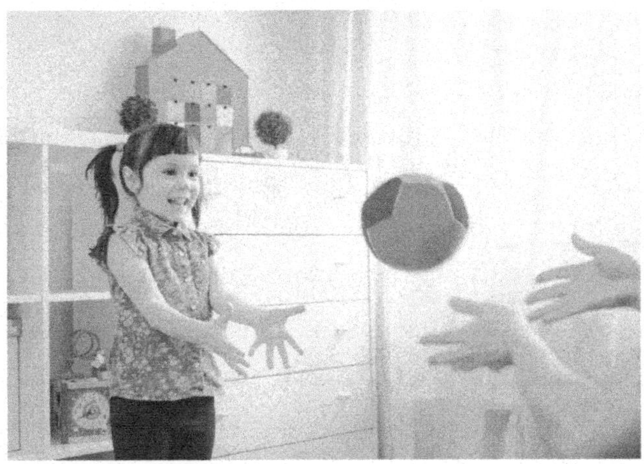

There are two types of practice that will help your child.

The first kind of practice is *focused* and *intentional*. Your child's speech pathologist will send practice assignments home. Pick a consistent time to practice before the child has an activity he enjoys. You may decide to practice before the child goes out to the park in the afternoon or before bath time each day. Your goal is to pay attention to the child's production of his sounds or words. You may need the child to face a mirror when practicing. Practice can be fun. Choose a toy to use between each correct production of the word. Some children enjoy tossing a basketball in a hoop or rolling a toy car down a ramp or getting playing the princess cupcake game and getting a piece of each cupcake. The idea is to have the child use the mirror and aim for correct production of each word. If he doesn't produce it correctly, try to gently ask him to try again and model the correct production of the sound. After each correct production, toss a basketball or add to the cupcake. Just don't let the game overwhelm the focus! Practice time does not have to be long. It is more important to practice consistently every day and aim for correct production. When practice time is over, move to the child's preferred activity, such as going to the park or taking a bath.

The second kind of practice is *generalization.* This is helping your child speak clearly in everyday life. For example, if your child is working on producing a /k/ sound and asks for a "too-tie," you can smile and say, "Oh, I hear your sound! Listen: *coo-kie!* Can you try to say *cookie?*" You are trying to help him generalize his skills on *sounds or words he has worked on in therapy.* If he cannot make a /k/ sound and is not yet working on it in speech therapy, this would not be appropriate to generalize yet.

Please do not "practice in the car." Quite a few parents are driving in traffic with their child buckled into a car seat in the back and they practice their speech sounds. This is not focused. You cannot make a left turn through an intersection while carefully looking in the mirror to check your child's mouth movements, and he cannot see you model the correct word!

The most important things to remember about practice are that concentrated, purposeful practice for just a few minutes every day is more effective than frantic practice "in the car" on the way to speech therapy!

CONCLUSION

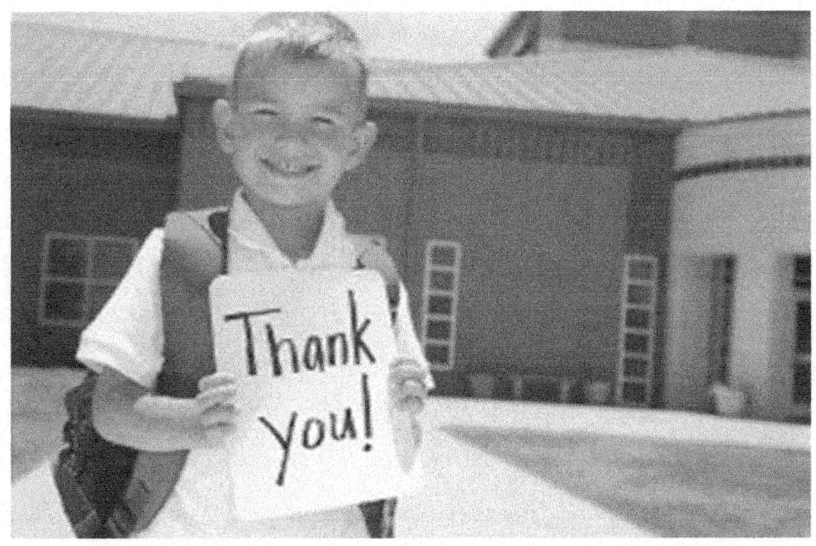

Watching your child grow is like watching a precious flower bud unfold, petal by petal. You anxiously observe each emerging petal. If you are reading this book, you are concerned because your child is not be speaking as you expected.

Remember, learning to speak is a natural process. Most children learn to speak without special instruction. If your child is *not* learning to speak naturally, it is important to find out *why* and take specific steps to help your child reach his maximum potential.

Sometimes, there are family situations that might make a parent feel uncomfortable about seeking a speech evaluation for a child. Would you feel better *knowing* if your child is on target or needs extra help?

Kate, the mother of Delta, said this beautifully: *It was very disheartening and discouraging to notice my child missing milestones that other children pass so easily. It felt like we were being left behind.*

When my daughter was a toddler, I noticed that she did not point to things like other children did. She did not reach her arms towards me and say "up." She was babbling cheerfully, but it was sing-song babbling with no real words. I had a thousand one-sided conversations with her, but I heard no real words from her.

To me, it didn't seem like there was anything "wrong" because she was so happy and bright. It was other women, mostly a group of aunties, who identified the problem because they had experienced a child like that in their own families.

What held me back the most was hearing people say, "Oh, she'll get it, she's just a late talker." That's anything but the truth. The late talker excuse was not a good one for me to hear because it just caused me to hesitate.

My advice to parents is that it's not about you, it's about the child. If you're hesitating to have a professional assess your child, just go for it – it couldn't hurt and it could only help. If you're a first-time parent, a professional could put you at ease by giving you pointers.

I have learned that I can't keep my daughter all to myself. I can't hesitate to provide her with something that could possibly benefit her. I have to do it. The best thing I've done for my daughter is to expose her to as many adults and positive influences as possible. She has met with so many professionals who give her love and attention and she deserves all of it.

References

Part I: Language

Acredolo, L., & Goodwyn, S. (1996). *Baby signs. How to talk to your baby before your baby can talk.* Chicago: NTB/ Contemporary.

Adamson, L.B. (2014). Joint Attention and Language Development. In Brooks, P.J. & Kempe, V. (eds.) Encyclopedia of Language Development, 299-303.

American Speech-Language-Hearing Association (2008). *Core Knowledge and Skills in Early Intervention.* Retrieved from www.asha.org/policy.

Bowen, C. (1998). Brown's Stages of Syntactic and Morphological Development. Retrieved from www.speech-language-therapy.com

Brown, R. (1973). *A first language: The early stages.* London: George Allen & Unwin.

C Yoshinaga-Itano, AL Sedey, DK Coulter, AL Mehl (1998) Language of early-and later-identified children with hearing loss. Pediatrics 102 (5), 1161-1171 1998

C Yoshinaga-Itano, ML Apuzzo, (1998) Identification of hearing loss after age 18 months is not early enough. American annals of the deaf, 380-387

Capone Singleton, N. & Shulman, B.B. (2019). 20Q: Language Development and Its Clinical Applications. *SpeechPathology.com,* Article 20088. Retrieved from www.speechpathology.com.

Capone Singleton, N. (2018). Late Talkers: Why the Wait-and-See Approach Is Outdated. *Pediatric Clinics of North America* on Pediatric Speech and Language: Perspectives on Inter-Professional Practice, 65(1), 13-29. https://doi.org/10.1016/j.pcl.2017.08.018

Capone Singleton, N., and Shulman, B. (2018). *Language Development. Foundations, Processes, and Clinical Applications.* 3nd Edition. Baltimore, MD: Jones & Bartlett Learning.

DiMitrova, N., Ozcaliskan, S., & Adamson, R.B. (2016). Parents' translations of child gestures facilitate word learning in children with autism, Down syndrome, and typical development. *Journal of Autism and Developmental Disorders, 46,* 221-231.

Gershkoff-Stowe, L., (2002). Object naming, vocabulary growth, and the development of word retrieval abilities. *Journal of Memory and Language, 46,* 665 – 687.

Hwa-Froelich, D. A. (2012). Childhood maltreatment and communication development. *Perspectives on school-based issues. 13*(1), 43-53.

Justice, Laura (2017, December) 20Q: Preventing Reading Difficulties in Children with Language Disorders. *SpeechPathology.com,* Article 19425. Retrieved from www.speechpathology.com

Krakower, Carol. Practical Theory of Mind Games – Learning Social Skills from the Bottom Up. Pro-Ed Publishers, 2013.

Lederer, Susan Hendler, PhD, CCC *Early Word Combinations: Assessment and Therapy Goals*

Lederer, Susan Hendler, PhD, CCC *Intervention – SW through Simple Sentences* - course presented on Medbridge, retrieved from www.medbridge.com

Lederer, Susan Hendler, PhD, CCC *The First Fifty Words* - course presented on Medbridge, retrieved from www.medbridge.com

Mandell, Jane, PhD, CCC/A . Back to Basics: Understanding Hearing Loss for Speech Pathologists Part I and Part II *Speech Pathology.com* Retrieved from www.speechpathology.com

McGregor, K.K., Rohlfing, K., Bean, A. & Marchner, E. (2009). Gesture as a Support for Word Learning: The Case of Under. *Journal of Child Language, 36*(4), 807-828.

McMurray, B. (2014). Neonatal speech perception. In Brooks, P.J. & Kempe, V. (eds.) Encyclopedia of Language Development, 576-580.

Miller, C.A. (2006). Developmental Relationships between Language and Theory of Mind, *American Journal of Speech-Language Pathology, 15*(2), 142-154.

Morise, Lacy, MS CCC-SLP and Sergent, Nicole MPT Ten Roadblocks to Natural Development *Medbridge,* 2014. Retrieved from <u>www.medbridge.com</u>

MP Moeller, JB Tomblin, C Yoshinaga-Itano, CMD Connor, S Jerger (2007) Current state of knowledge: Language and literacy of children with hearing impairment. Ear and hearing 28 (6), 740-753 2007

Paparella, T., Stickles Goods, K., Freeman, S., Kasari, C. (2011). The emergence of nonverbal joint attention and requesting skills in young children with autism. *Journal of Communication Disorders,* 44, 569-583.

Peak, Alison D, LCSW, IMH-E *The Role of Relationships in Early Development: The Connection Between Experiences and Language Capacity* – course presented by SpeechPathology.com

Rescorla, L. (1989). The Language Development Survey: A screening tool for delayed language in toddlers. *Journal of Speech and Hearing Disorders,54,* 587-599.

Sharma, A., Nash, A. A., and Dorman, M. (2009). Cortical development, plasticity and re-organization in children with cochlear implants. *J. Commun. Disord.* 42, 272–279. doi: 10.1016/j.jcomdis.2009.03.003

Tomasello (1995). Joint attention as social cognition. In Moore & Dunham (Eds.) Joint attention: Its origins and role in development. Hillsdale, NJ

Tomblin and Nippold (2014) Understanding Individual Differences in Language Development Across the School Years. Psychology Press.

Werker, J.F., Yeung, H.H., & Yoshida, K. (2012). How do infants become native speech perception experts? Current Directions in Psychological Science, 21(4), 221-226.

Part II: Speech

Bishop, D., Holt, G., Line, E. et al. (2012). Parental phonological memory contributes to prediction of outcome of late talkers from 20 months to 4 years: A longitudinal study of precursors of specific language impairment. *Journal of NeuroDevelopmental Disorders, 4:3.*

Davis, Barbara L., PhD, CCC-SLP *Goal and Target Selection for Early Vocal Development: Children Aged 0-3* – Course presented on Medbridge

Jakielski, Kathy J. PhD, CCC-SLP *Foundations for Clinical Practice: Vocal-to-Verbal Development* – course presented on Medbridge

Landau, B., Smith, L. B., & Jones, S.S. (1988). The importance of shape in early lexical learning. *Cognitive Development, 3,* 299-321.

Allen, M. M. (2013). Intervention efficacy and intensity for children with speech sound disorders. *Journal of Speech, Language and Hearing Research, 56,* 865-877.

American Speech-Language-Hearing Association. (2007). *Childhood apraxia of speech* [Technical Report]. Available from www.asha.org/policy.

Back to Basics: Foundations for CAS Interventions by Joleen R. Ferald, PhD, CCC-SLP, BCS-CL, speechpathology.com

Bislick, Lauren, PhD, CCC-SLP *Principles of Learning and Motor Speech Disorders* – course presented by Medbridge

Cabbage, K. L., Farquharson, K., Iuzzini-Seigel, J., Zuk, J., & Hogan, T. P. (2018). Exploring the overlap between dyslexia and speech sound production deficits. *Language, Speech, and Hearing Services in Schools, 49*(4), 774-786.

Carrigg, B., Parry, L., Baker, E., Shriberg, L. D., & Ballard, K. J. (2016). Cognitive, Linguistic, and Motor Abilities in a Multigenerational Family with Childhood Apraxia of Speech. *Archives of Clinical Neuropsychology, 31*(8), 1006-1025.

Caspari, S. (2007). Working Guidelines for the Assessment and Treatment of Childhood Apraxia of Speech: A Review of ASHA's 2007 Position Statement and Technical Report. http://www.speechpathology.com/articles/article_detail.asp?article_id=328

Davis, B. L., & Velleman, S. L. (2000). Differential diagnosis and treatment of developmental apraxia of speech in infants and toddlers. *Infant-Toddler Intervention, 10*, 177-192.

Davis, B. L., & Velleman, S. L. (2000). Differential diagnosis and treatment of developmental apraxia of speech in infants and toddlers. *Infant-Toddler Intervention, 10*, 177-192.

Delaney, A. L., & Kent, R. D. (2004, November). Developmental profiles of children diagnosed with apraxia of speech. Poster session presented at the annual convention of the American-Speech-Language-Hearing Association, Philadelphia.

Dodd, B., Hua, Z., Crosbie, S., Holm, A., & Ozanne, A. (2006). *Diagnostic Evaluation of Articulation and Phonology (DEAP).* Pearson Education, Inc.

Edeal, D. M. and Gildersleeve-Neumann, C. E. (2011). The importance of production frequency in therapy for childhood apraxia of speech, *American Journal of Speech-Language Pathology, 20*, 95-110. doi:10.1044/1058-0360(2011/09-0005)

Farnham, Teresa, MA, CCC-SLP Writing Simple Goals and Evaluating Progress Simply for Severe Phonological Disorders *Speech Pathology. com 2019,* retrieved from www.speechpathology.com

Farnham, Teresa, MA, CCC-SLP Complexity Theory and Effective Treatment Decisions for Severe Phonological Disorders. *SpeechPathology.com* 2019. Retrieved from www.speechpathology.com

Farquharson, Kelly PhD, CC-SLP *Connections Between Speech Sound Production and Literacy Skills* – recorded July 11, 2019 and presented on SpeechPathology.com

Fernard, Joleen R., PhD, CCC-SLP, BCS-CL Back to Basics: Foundations for CAS Intervention. *Speech Pathology.com.* 2019. Retrieved from www.speechpathology.com

Fish, M. (2016). *Here's How to Treat Childhood Apraxia of Speech-Second Edition.* San Diego, CA., Plural Publishing Inc.

Frameword for Differential Diagnosis of Pediatric Motor Speech Disorders - *Medbridge course, Edyth Strand*

Golding-Kushner, K.J. (2018). 20Q: Velo-Cardio-Facial Syndrome (VCFS). *SpeechPathology.com,* Article 19904. Retrieved from www.speechpathology.com

Hammer, D. & Stoeckel, R. (2006). *A comparison of childhood apraxia of speech, dysarthria, and severe phonological disorder.* Childhood Apraxia of Speech Association of North America (CASANA). Retrieved August 4, 2018 from http://www.apraxia-kids.org/library/a-comparison-of-childhood-apraxia-of-speech-dysarthria-and-severe-phonological-disorder/

Hayden, D., Namasivayam, A. K. & Ward, R. (2015) The assessment of fidelity in a motor speech-treatment approach, *Speech, Language and Hearing,* 18:1, 30-38, DOI: 10.1179/2050572814Y.0000000046

Hodson, B. (2004). *Hodson Assessment of Phonological Patterns-Third Edition (HAPP-3).* Oceanside, CA. Academic Communication Associates, Inc.

Hodson, Barbara Williams, PhD *Evaluating and Enhancing Children's Phonological Systems* – course presented on SpeechPathology.com

Journal of the American Dental Association: https://jada.ada.org/article/S0002-8177(14)61211-3/fulltext

Kummer, Ann W. PhD, CCC-SLP *Evaluation and Treatment of Speech/ Resonance Disorders and Velopharyngeal Dysfunction - course* presented on SpeechPathology.com

LaSalle, Lisa R., PhD, CCC-SLP *Updates in Phonological Process Analysis in Preschoolers* – course presented by SpeechPathology.com

Lewis, B. A., Freebairn, L. A., Hansen, A. J., Iyengar, S.K., & Taylor, H. G. (2004). School –age follow-up of children with childhood apraxia of speech. *Language, Speech, and Hearing Services in Schools, 35:* 122-140.

McCormack, J., McAllister, L. McLeod, S. & Harrison, L. J., (2012). Knowing, having, doing: The battles of childhood speech impairment. *Child Language Teaching and Therapy, 28,* 141–157.

McLeod, S., & Baker, E. (2017). *Children's speech: An evidence-based approach to assessment and intervention.* Boston, MA:

McNeill B. C., Wolter J. and Gillon, G.T. (2017) A comparison of the metalinguistic performance and spelling development of children with inconsistent speech sound disorder and their age-matched and reading-matched peers. *American Journal of Speech-Language Pathology, 26, 456-468.*

Millington, Marnie, MS, CCC-SLP *Assessment of Young Children with Suspected CAS* – course presented on Medbridge

Moriarty, B. & Gillon, G. (2006). Phonological awareness intervention or children with childhood apraxia of speech. *International Journal of Language & Communication Disorders,*42 (6), 713-734.

Murray, E., McCabe, P., & Ballard, K. J. (2014). A systematic review of treatment outcomes for children with childhood apraxia of speech. *American Journal of Speech-Language Pathology, 17,* 1-19.

Murray, E., McCabe, P., & Ballard, K. J. (2015). A randomized controlled trial for children with childhood apraxia of speech comparing rapid syllable transition treatment and the Nuffield Dyspraxia

Programme–third edition, *Journal of Speech, Language, and Hearing Research*, June 2015, Vol. 58, 669-686.

Namasivayam, A. K., Pukonen, M., Goshulak, D., Yu.V.Y., Kadis, D.S., Kroll, R., Pang, E.W., & De Nil, L.F. (2013). Changes in speech intelligibility following motor speech treatment in children. *Journal of Communication Disorders*, 46(3):264-80.

Newmeyer, A. J., Aylward, C., Akers, R., Ishikawa, K., Grether, S., deGrauw, T., Grasha C. and White, J. (2009). Results of the sensory profile in children with suspected childhood apraxia of speech. *Physical & Occupational Therapy in Pediatrics, 29, (2), 203-218.*

Nijland, L., Terband, H. and Maassen, B., (20015) Cognitive Functions in Childhood Apraxia of Speech *Journal of Speech, Language, and Hearing Research, 58, 550–565.*

Overby, M. and Caspari, S. (2015). Volubility, consonant, and syllable characteristics in infants and toddlers later diagnosed with childhood apraxia of speech; A pilot study. *Journal of Communication Disorders, 55, 44-62.*

Peter, B. & Stoel-Gammon, C. (2008). Central timing disorders in subtypes of primary speech disorders. *Clinical Linguistics & Phonetics, 22* (3) 171-198.

Shriberg, L. D. (2010). Childhood speech sound disorders: From post-behaviourism to the postgenomic era. In R. Paul & P. Flipsen Jr. (Eds.), *Speech sound disorders in children: In honour of Lawrence D. Shriberg* (pp. 1–33). San Diego, CA: Plural Publishing.

Shriberg, L. D., Kwiatkowski, J., & Mabie, H. L. (2019). Estimates of the prevalence of motor speech disorders in children with idiopathic speech delay. *Clinical Linguistics and Phonetics*, 1-28.

Shriberg, L. D., Potter, N. A., & Strand, E., A. (2009). Childhood apraxia of speech in children and adolescents with Galactosemia.

Skinder-Meredith, A. (2017, October). 20Q: Childhood Apraxia of Speech (CAS): Diagnosis and Treatment.

SpeechPathology.com, Article 19340. Retrieved from www.speechpathology.com.

Stackhouse, J. (1997). Phonological awareness: Connecting speech and literacy problems. In B. Hodson and M.L. Edwards (Eds.), *Perspectives in Applied Phonology* (pp. 157-196). Gaithersburg, MD: Aspen Publications.

Strand, E. A., & Skinder, A. (1999). Treatment of developmental apraxia of speech: Integral stimulation methods. In A. J. Caruso and E. A. Strand, (Eds.) *Clinical Management of Motor Speech Disorders of Children.* New York: Thieme Publishing Co.

Strand, E. A., McCauley, R. J., Weigand, S. D., Stoeckel, R. E., & Bass, B. S. (2013). A motor speech assessment for children with severe speech disorders: Reliability and validity evidence. *Journal of Speech, Language, and Hearing Research, 56,* 505-520.

Strand, E., Stoeckel, R., & Baas, B (2006.) Treatment of severe childhood apraxia of speech: A treatment efficacy study. *Journal of Medical Speech-Language Pathology, 14*(4), 297-307.

Sugden, E., Baker, E., Munro, N., Williams, A. L., & Trivette, C. M. (2018). Service delivery and intervention intensity for phonology-based speech sound disorders. *International Journal of Language and Communication Disorders, 53*(4), 718-734.

Warren, S. F., Fey, M. E., & Yoder, P. J. (2007). Differential treatment intensity research: A missing link to creating optimally effective communication interventions. *Mental Retardation and Developmental Disabilities Research Reviews, 13,* 70-77.

Williams, A. L. (2012). Intensity in phonological intervention: Is there a prescribed amount? *International Journal of Speech-Language Pathology, 14*(5), 456-461.

Williams, A. Lynn and Baker, Elise. 20Q: Speech Sound Disorders in Children: What's New? *SpeechPathology.com, Retrieved* from www.speechpathology.com.

Stuttering:

Ambrose, N. G., Yairi, E., Loucks, T. M., Seery, C. H., & Throneburg, R. (2015). Relation of motor, linguistic and temperament factors in epidemiologic subtypes of persistent and recovered stuttering: Initial findings. *Journal of fluency disorders, 45,* 12-26.

Bernstein Ratner, N. (1997). Stuttering: A psycholinguistic perspective. In R.F. Curlee and G. Siegel (Eds.). *Nature and treatment of stuttering: New directions* (2nd ed.). (pp. 97-127). Needham Heights, MA: Allyn & Bacon.

Boey, R.A., Van de Heyning, P.H., Wuyts, F.L., Heylen, L., Stoop, R., & De Bodt, M.S. (2009). Awareness and reactions of young stuttering children aged 2-7 years old towards their speech disfluency. *Journal of Communication Disorders, 42,* 344-346.

Chang, S. E., Angstadt, M., Chow, H. M., Etchell, A. C., Garnett, E. O., Choo, A. L., & Sripada, C. (2017). Anomalous network architecture of the resting brain in children who stutter. *Journal of Fluency Disorders.*

Chang, S-E. (2014). Research Updates in Neuroimaging Studies of Children Who Stutter. *Seminars in Speech and Language, 35,* 67–79.

Constantino, C., Leslie, P., Quesal, R.W., & Yaruss, J.S. (2016). Day-to-day variability of stuttering. *Journal of Communication Disorders, 60,* 39-50.

Costello, J.M. & Ingham, R.J. (1984). Assessment strategies for stuttering. In R.F. Curlee, & W.H. Perkins (Eds.), *Nature and treatment of stuttering: new directions.* San Diego: College-Hill Press.

Craig Coleman: Risk Factors for Young Children Who Stutter – course on Speech Pathology.com

Ezrati-Vinacour, R., Platzky, R., & Yairi, E. (2001). The young child's awareness of stuttering-like disfluency. *Journal of Speech, Language, and Hearing Research, 44,* 368-80.

Felsenfeld, S., Kirk, K.M., Zhu, G., Statham, D.J., Neale, M.C., Martin, N.G. (2000). A study of the genetic and environmental etiology of stuttering in a selected twin sample. *Behavioral Genetics, 30*(5), 359–366.

Frigerio-Domingues, Carlos & Drayna, Dennis. Genetic contributions to stuttering: the current evidence. Molecular Genetics & Genomic Medicine, Volume 5, Issue 2, March 2017 p. 93-184

Hitti, S. (2016). *Implications of Effortful Control and Negative Affectivity in the Persistence and Recovery of Stuttering* (Doctoral dissertation, Vanderbilt University).

Johnson, W. (1941, April). An Open Letter to the mother of a "Stuttering" Child. *You and Your Child.* (Reprinted in 1949 in the *Journal of Speech and Hearing Disorders, 14,* 3-18.

Jones, R., Choi, D., Conture, E.G., & Walden, T. (2015). Temperament, emotion, and childhood stuttering. *Seminars in Speech and Language, 35,* 114-131.

Kelly, E. (2017, April). Vanderbilt SLP Journal Club: Differentiating Stuttering Persistence and Recovery. *SpeechPathology.com,* Article 19082. Retrieved from: http://www.speechpathology.com..

Kraft, S.J., & Yairi, E. (2011). Genetic Bases of Stuttering: The State of the Art, 2011. *Folia Phoniatrica et Logopaedica, 64,* 34-47.

Langevin, M., Packman, A., & Onslow, M. (2009). Peer responses to stuttering in the preschool setting. *American Journal of Speech-Language Pathology, 18,* 264-276.

Langevin, M., Packman, A., & Onslow, M. (2010). Parent perceptions of the impact of stuttering on their preschoolers and themselves. *Journal of Communication Disorders, 43,* 407-423.

Manning, W. (2010). *Clinical decision making in fluency disorders* (3rd ed.). Clifton Park, NY: Delmar, Cengage Learning.

Månsson H. (2000). Childhood stuttering: Incidence and development. *Journal of Fluency Disorders, 25,* 47–57.

Mohan, R., & Weber, C. (2015). Neural systems mediating processing of sound units of language distinguish recovery versus persistence in stuttering. *Journal of neurodevelopmental disorders, 7*(1), 28.

Moore, S.E., & Perkins, W.H. (1990). Validity and reliability of judgments of authentic and simulated stuttering. *Journal of Speech and Hearing Disorders, 55,* 383-391.

Perkins, W.H. (1990). What is stuttering? *Journal of Speech and Hearing Disorders, 55,* 379-382.

Reardon-Reeves, N., & Yaruss, J.S. (2013). *School-age stuttering therapy: A practical guide.* McKinney, TX: Stuttering Therapy Resources, Inc.

Reilly, S., Onslow, M., Packman, A., Cini, E., Conway, L., Ukoumunne, O.C., et al. (2013). Natural history of stuttering to 4 years of age: a prospective community-based study. *Pediatrics, 132*(3), 460–467.

Riley, G., & Riley, J. (1986). Oral-motor discoordination among children who stutter. *Journal of Fluency Disorders, 11,* 335-344.

Shapiro, D. (2011). Stuttering intervention: A collaborative journey to fluency freedom. (2nd ed.). Austin, TX: Pro-Ed.

Spencer, C. & Weber-Fox, C. (2014). Preschool speech articulation and nonword repetition abilities may help predict eventual recovery or persistence of stuttering. *Journal of Fluency Disorders, 41,* 32-46.

St. Louis, K.O., & Hinzman, A. (1988). A descriptive study of speech, language, and hearing characteristics of school-age stutterers. *Journal of Fluency Disorders, 13,* 331-355.

Usler, E., & Weber-Fox, C. (2015). Neurodevelopment for syntactic processing distinguishes childhood stuttering recovery versus persistence. *Journal of Neurodevelopmental Disorders, 7:4.*

Usler, E., Smith, A., & Weber, C. (2017). A lag in speech motor coordination during sentence production is associated with stuttering persistence in young children. *Journal of Speech, Language, and Hearing Research, 60,* 51-61.

Vanryckeghem, M., Brutten, G.J., & Hernandez, L.M. (2005). A comparative investigation of the speech-associated attitude of preschool and kindergarten children who do and do not stutter. *Journal of Fluency Disorders, 30,* 307-318.

Yairi, E. (1997). Disfluency characteristics of childhood stuttering. In R. Curlee & G. Siegel (Eds.). *Nature and treatment of stuttering: New Directions* (2nd ed.) (pp. 49-78). Boston: Allyn & Bacon.

Yairi, E., & Ambrose, N. (1992a). A longitudinal study of stuttering in children: A preliminary report. *Journal of Speech and Hearing Research, 35,* 755-760.

Yairi, E., & Ambrose, N. (1992b). Onset of stuttering in preschool children: Selected factors. *Journal of Speech and Hearing Research, 35,* 782-788.

Yairi, E., & Ambrose, N. (1999). Early childhood stuttering I: Persistency and recovery rates. *Journal of Speech Language and Hearing Research, 42,* 1097-1112.

Yairi, E., & Ambrose, N. (2013). Epidemiology of stuttering: 21st century advances. *Journal of Fluency Disorders, 38*(2), 66–87.

Yaruss, J.S. & Reardon-Reeves, N. (2017, May). 20Q: Early Childhood Stuttering: Background and Assessment. *SpeechPathology.com,* Article 19130. Retrieved from www.speechpathology.com

Yaruss, J.S. (1997a). Clinical measurement of stuttering behaviors. *Contemporary Issues in Communication Science and Disorders, 24,* 33-44.

Yaruss, J.S. (1997b). Clinical implications of situational variability in preschool children who stutter. *Journal of Fluency Disorders, 22,* 187-203.

Yaruss, J.S. (1998). Describing the consequences of disorders: Stuttering and the International Classification of Impairments, Disabilities, and Handicaps. *Journal of Speech, Language, and Hearing Research, 49,* 249-257.